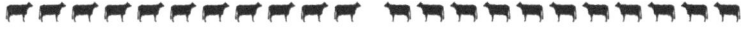

HANDBOOK *for*

BEEF CALF HEALTH

Bob Sager, DVM PhD DABVP

Handbook for Beef Calf Health
R.B. (Bob) Sager DVM PhD DABVP (Beef Cattle)

Medicine Creek Bovine Health Solutions and Consulting
441 Daisy Dean Road
Wilsall, Montana 59086
hammerbeef.sager97@gmail.com
www.MedicineCreekBovineHealth.com

Produced by IndieBookLauncher.com
Cover Design: Saul Bottcher
Interior Design and Typesetting: Saul Bottcher
The body text of this book is set in Adobe Jenson.

Formats Available
Paperback ISBN 978-1-77342-055-4
Hardcover ISBN 978-1-77342-056-1
EPUB ISBN 978-1-77342-057-8
Kindle ISBN 978-1-77342-058-5

CONTENTS

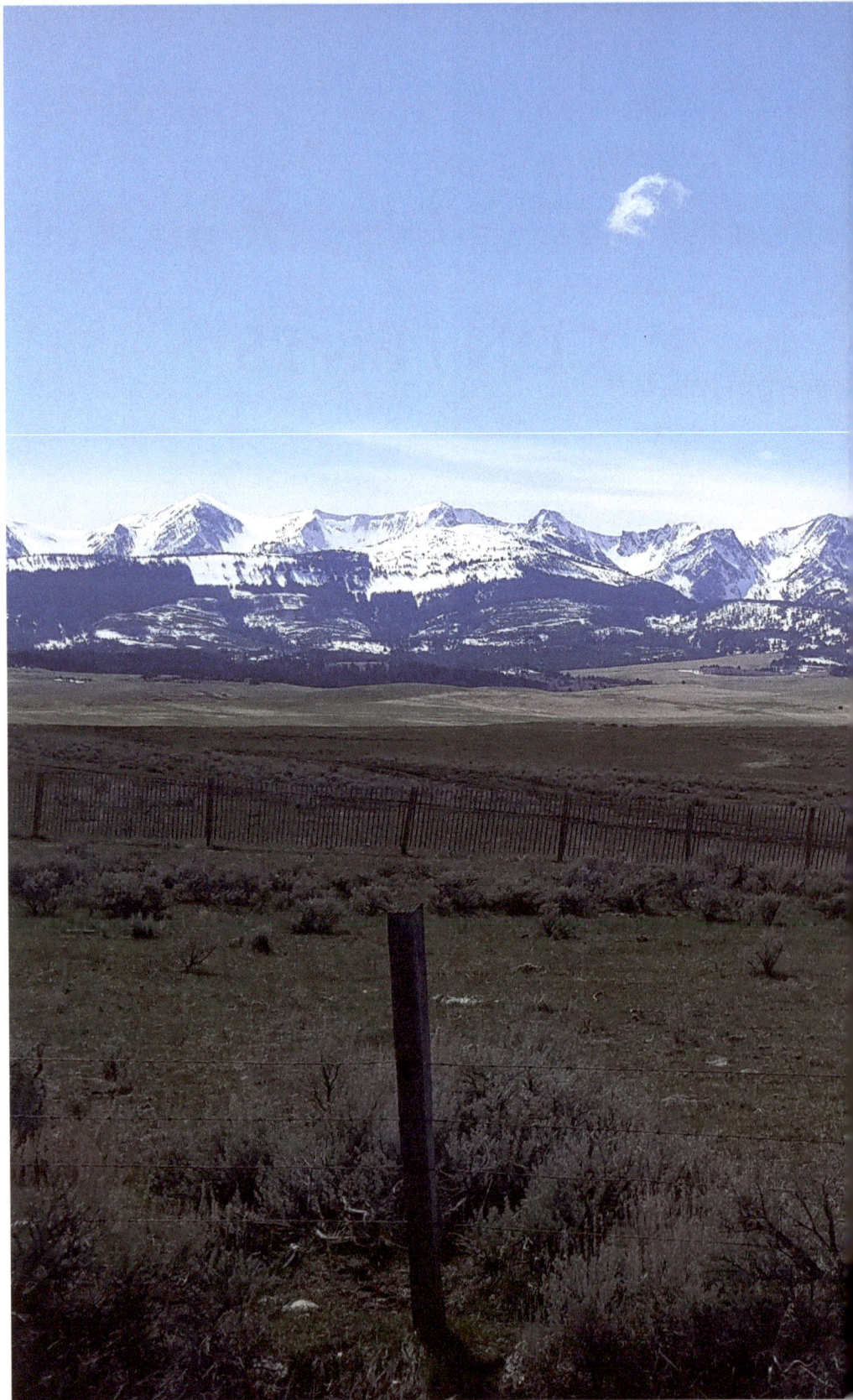

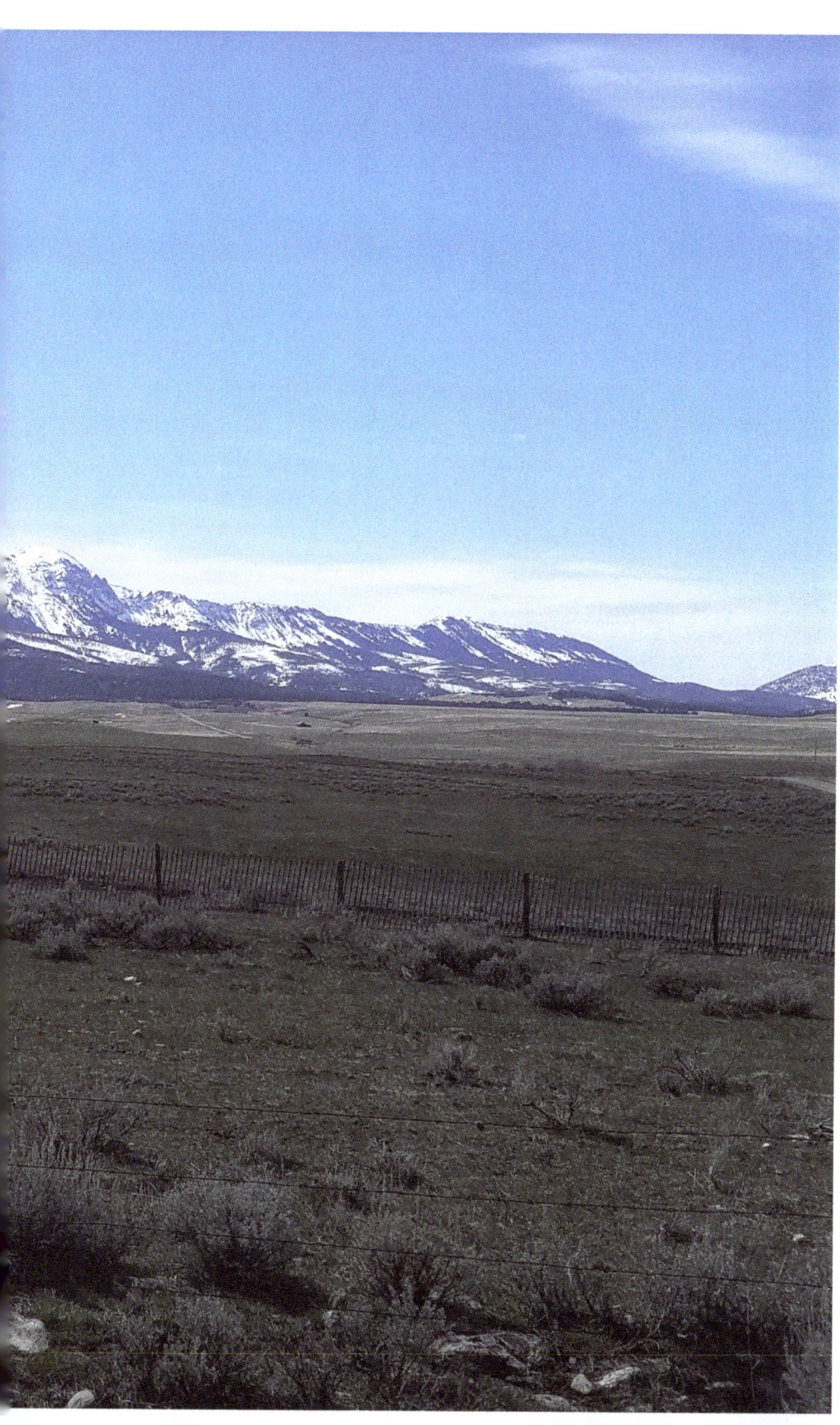

Preface

This book is dedicated to the rancher who, each day, defies odds by enduring challenges of weather, economics, labor, and animal health to produce the world's finest beef in an environment that is both harsh and beautiful. Few labors of life are as demanding of labor, as requiring of toleration of weather and environment, as challenging in combining science with management, and as fulfilling and rewarding as beef cattle production. For those that are blessed to live where they choose and work the career they desire: this book is dedicated to those "modern cowboys" who work in the shadow of those before them and lead the way for those following in the beef cattle industry.

This handbook is also dedicated to my father, H.B. Sager, who introduced me to cattle production at an early age and guided me to understand the challenges and rewards of beef cattle production. He also encouraged me to continue the legacy of a sixth-generation family in beef cattle production. The reflections he shared with his son were of the enjoyment of being around cattle, the demanding importance of good animal husbandry, and the life of being a "cowboy in Montana". My father entered Colorado A & M (presently Colorado State University) in 1921 to study veterinary medicine, only to be called back to the ranch at La Veta, Colorado to help his ill father run the ranch. He never made it back to school but lived his life as a rancher and helped me in my veterinary practices for nearly twenty years at Belgrade and Wilsall, Montana. I am proud of my heritage and proud that my father introduced me to beef cattle production, therefore, this handbook is dedicated to his memory and his love for beef cattle production.

This handbook began as a project to fulfill partial requirements for a Master of Science, Animal and Range Sciences, Montana State

University, graduate degree under the advisement and guidance of John Paterson PhD. During the 42 years as a practicing veterinarian in Montana, I was constantly interested in learning more about the interaction of nutrition and the bovine immune system. While as a practicing veterinarian I was continually learning about the importance of nutrition in beef cattle production, I also desired to continue my formal educational journey in learning more about the important interactions of minerals with bovine health. Therefore, I decided to continue my education and started graduate school, with a focus on micro-mineral nutrition affecting the immune system in beef cattle production.

My focus while attending graduate school was to understand the interaction of the element cobalt (Co) on the immune system of beef calves. This journey started many years ago with a desire to answer a question that arose before, doing field investigation work for animal health companies, in evaluating vaccine failure problems in my practice area during my career. During my graduate program, I completed research evaluating the effects of different levels of cobalt supplementation (above National Research Council recommended levels) and the response of the bovine immune system in weaned beef calves. Many vaccine failure problems were primary copper (Cu) deficiency problems, due to antagonistic interactions with iron (Fe), molybdenum (Mo), and sulfates (SO_4) in the drinking water. While the primary problem was copper, most of the vaccine failure problems had underlining cobalt deficiencies at the same time. Reviewing literature and research articles indicated there was no information on cobalt influencing the immune system in beef cattle.

Personally, I had a goal to continue my education after selling my practice and enrolled at Montana State University in the fall of 2009, finishing with a Master's in Animal and Range Sciences (under advising by John Paterson, PhD) in May of 2011. As stated, this handbook was a graduate project that was the idea of Dr. Paterson, to be used by Montana County Extension Agents, Montana ranchers, and students in beef production as a guide to help understand the basics of beef calf health from birth to weaning at six-to-eight months of age.

The major objective of this Handbook is to describe, with the aid of images, charts, graphs and diagrams, the importance of beef calf health during the first 6-8 months of life. Wherever possible, graphs and diagrams have been used to help the reader to better visualize the important concepts, and thus hopefully fulfilling the need for a practical and concise handbook that will present beef calf health in "cowboy language", to be used by ranchers, students, and county extension agents. The purpose of this handbook is not to be used as a reference text, but for a concise source of information for beef calf health management, specific major diseases, colostrum importance and feeding, and an informative source for concepts important to health and economic return in beef cattle production.

This handbook is divided into chapters based on beef calf health concepts for successful production applicable to ranchers and students that are interested in improving beef calf health. Chapters are divided in a chronological period of calf growth and when the producer will recognize these important challenges and problems. Chapters written inform the producer of the problem, how to correct or treat the problem, and a recommendation for solution or recommendation of management to prevent the problem for occurring.

Much of this handbook is based on experiences and knowledge gained from a personal career in beef cattle production medicine by the author, while other portions are based on experiences and health concepts that were addressed by clients during a forty-plus-year career in bovine production medicine.

I have made an effort to write a take-home message with each major concept. Present times are exciting in the beef industry due to recent increases in demand and consumer price, yet production costs continue to present challenges requiring more emphasis on management and a greater demand on proper nutrition. The excitement is often lowered with the industry having a history of continued cyclic troubled times. We must understand that we as producers are still highly influenced by the consumer who demands high-quality beef that is raised under strict health and welfare conditions.

After the initial writing of the Handbook for Beef Calf Heath, I worked at the University of Missouri College of Veterinary Medicine and started my PhD. I completed my doctorate (PhD) in Animal Science and taught animal science classes at Montana State University before being employed by Miratorg Holdings / Bryansk Meat Company near Bryansk, Russia for more than twenty -two months as the senior veterinarian. During this time, I saw the expansion of the corporation to 57 farms: 34 cow-calf units, 23 yearling or replacement operations, and two feedlots with a capacity of over 125,000 head.

This project is the world's largest vertical integrated beef cattle complex, including over 437,000 head of Angus beef cattle. This gave me an excellent opportunity to utilize the principles of this Handbook, and to see first hand the success of a proper diagnosis, implementation of sound management toward proper treatment, and the importance of the basic understanding of cattle behavior and proper animal husbandry for optimum performance and health.

This opportunity also reflected what can happen without proper care, deficiency of minimum nutrition, and how critical the basic understanding of proper beef cattle welfare, low-stress handling, and skilled experienced labor is to performance and health in a large beef cattle operation. America's beef cattle industry is blessed to have skilled, knowledgeable, caring operators that have grown up in the beef cattle industry, that understand the importance of proper husbandry, basic requirements of nutrition, and how beef cattle welfare all affect performance and health toward profit. The rest of the world is learning this as we have the past one hundred years.

Introduction

This handbook has been written in "cowboy language" and is meant to be a quick reference guide for many of the common questions and challenges associated with beef calf production. The book provides a written take-home message on each topic.

United States beef production has changed significantly in the past fifty years, mostly through the application of technology and improved genetics. Along with the rapid transition from small herd production (operations with fewer than 100 head of cattle) to larger ranch operations and the growth of 100,000-head corporate-owned feedlots, there has been vast use of new technologies that include improved use of genetics, increased nutrition, refined implant usage, and the employment of new vaccine management for improved health and increased performance during production.

With the use of improved forage and grain genetics, feed production has greatly increased, resulting in beef production costs decreasing and beef production efficiency increasing. This has helped to keep beef prices lower and has increased the market share for beef, compared to other protein choices, over the past twenty years.

Commercial beef slaughter has decreased by 16% since 1975, yet total beef production has increased by 10% (Wileman and Thomson, 2008). In the same time the carcass weights have increased by over 25% (Paterson, 2009), so the total weight of four steers today exceeds the weight of five steers just over thirty years ago. These trends seem to be continuing. The carcass weights have increased by 190 lb. (86.3 kg) from carcass weights in the 1970's, meanwhile cow numbers have decreased by 30% over the same period. Most of this has been because of the increased efficiency of beef production and this trend will continue in the future. Few industries can boast of such great strides in production efficiency as the United States beef industry.

Beef and cattle prices increased to record levels just prior to the writing of this Handbook (over the period 2011-2014) and are expected to push even higher in the next few years. Several years of declining cattle inventories culminated in late 2011 with a projected 3% decrease in slaughter that combined with lighter carcass weights to result in 3.8% less beef in the fourth quarter of 2011 compared to the previous year. During 2012, slaughter dropped by another 5%, even with an increase in carcass weights.

As of the writing of this book, we are in the most "bullish market seen in the history of beef production", as calf prices have set an all-time high.

Decreasing numbers will influence steady increases in price. Weather in the Southwest United States in 2011 and 2012 dramatically dropped cow numbers in the southern plain states and contributed to a decreased supply and continued to influence supply levels for the next few years. As with most consumer-driven commodities, supply is the main factor in recently pushing prices higher. Consumer demand for beef is a combination of willingness and ability to purchase a given quantity of a product at a given price. However, beef as a product reflects differences in consumer demands; and when demands are increased there also occur changes in different beef products being developed. Questions on whether consumer preferences have changed along with increasing prices will determine the beef products desired. Recently, ground beef demand continues to grow, including demand for premium ground beef products. The industry will need to change and adjust in relation to changes in consumer demand in the future.

With the emerging awareness of animal welfare, another intent of this handbook is to help the reader make better decisions toward improving beef calf health, and to recommend increased general animal welfare principals for producing beef calves. Animal welfare is the responsibility of all of us in beef production, and as society demands increasing awareness and action towards improving animal welfare, we as producers must assume a larger role in this important area. A pro-active stance is doing production in a way that benefits both animal and man.

The world is developing a desire for beef, because of the increasing population that now has access to beef and has gained a desire for the taste and nutritional advantages that beef provides compared to other protein foods. The economy of the world has grown, allowing the world's population to purchase beef products and experience the desired flavor and taste. It is believed this trend will continue, allowing beef production to expand and provide a positive economic return for those in the beef cattle industry. Future experiences in beef cattle production may provide good economic returns along with the "romance" experienced by past generations. Truly this is an exciting time in the beef cattle industry, resulting from the use of improved genetics, application of new animal health technologies, and the efficient use of management and animal welfare in producing the world's finest beef.

In my career I had the opportunity to interact with many successful ranchers with diverse ranching operations. However, those that were the most successful had these common traits:

1. They were passionate about beef production and they enjoyed every aspect of the ranching operation.

2. They interacted with their veterinarian or animal health specialist, read current information to update their knowledge, or attended animal health education meetings or workshops. I personally had a difficult time keeping ahead of what they read or knew in terms of new or updated technology.

3. They practiced good animal husbandry by keeping their operation clean and up-to-date, practiced humane animal care, were conservative in buying equipment, and accepted new technology to be included in their ranch operation.

4. The most successful often were the ones that practiced the best range management, implemented care in stocking rates, and always planned ahead for next year in pasture and feed assets. Use of natural windbreaks in brush and creek-bottom feeding during weather stress periods were used to create better animal comfort away from wind chill factors. Continually improving water use and pasture use was a priority. They were excellent stewards of the land.

5. Those that were most successful economically had moderately-sized cows and the calf weaned per body weight of the

cow was the highest. They also had the highest rate of calves weaned per cows exposed and did not over-feed cows during the winter months. Many used pasture during the winter months, fed a small percent of straw to lower feed costs after meeting National Research Council requirements, and were careful in evaluating mineral intake by their cows during the year.

6. It seemed like the most successful ranchers were always the most happy and optimistic with life in general. They balanced family, faith, and work.

7. All were proud to be ranchers, serving in America's Agriculture Production. As a result, they were great Ambassadors of the "Cowboy Life".

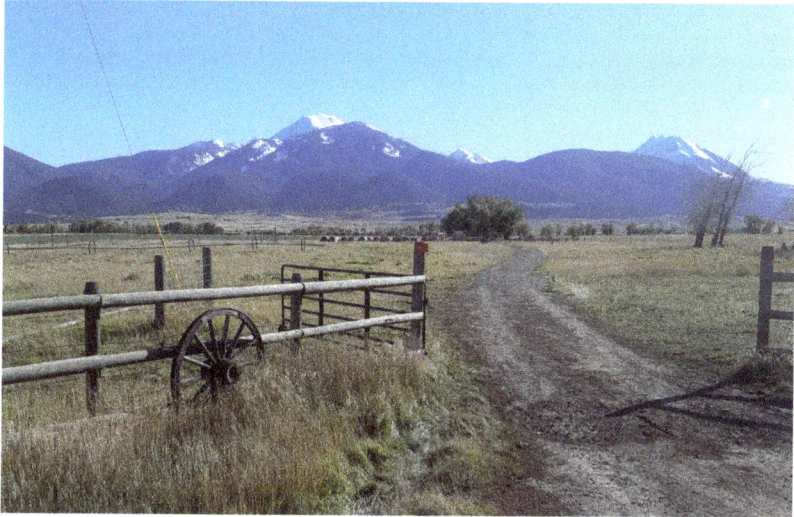

1

Gestational Nutrition and Care

Normal calf health starts almost one year before the birth of the calf. Even the conception process is a result of the proper nutrition and body weight gain necessary to activate the hormonal processes required for estrous and fertilization.

Gestational Nutrition

Gestational nutrition is vital for the survival and development of the fetus. A balance of proteins, carbohydrates, minerals, vitamins, and lipids are required. Meeting nutrient requirements, especially for proteins and especially during late gestation, is also essential to ensure quality and quantity of colostrum, the most important nutrient for the newborn calf.

The following table summarizes some nutrient requirements of lactating and pregnant beef cows.

Nutrient	Lactating cows	Pregnant cows
Protein (% of ration)	9.5–12.5%	7.0–9.0%
Protein (lbs/day)	1.8–2.9 lbs.	1.1–1.8 lbs.
Total Digestible Nutrients (TDN) %	55–69%	49–64%
TDN lbs/day	10.5–17.0 lbs.	8.0–13.0 lbs.
Metabolized energy (calories / lb. ration)	0.9–1.3 Mcal	0.8–1.1 Mcal
Metabolized energy (calories / day)	0.25–0.50 Mcal	0.20–0.30 Mcal
Ca & P (grams/day)	25–40 g	15–25 g

Table 1: Nutrient requirements for lactation and gestation of moderate-framed beef cows.[1]

Body condition scores

The Body Condition Score (BCS) of cows before calving is critical for beef calf success. It is well established that BCS of cows at calving is related to reproductive performance.[2]

Research has found that BCS of cows at the time of calving is the most reliable factor that can be used to predict whether cows will be-

1.   Data from *Animal Feeding and Nutrition, 9th Edition*, Marshall H. Jurgens.
2.   Wiltbank et al., 1962; Dunn and Kaltenbach, 1980; Richards et al., 1986, Selk et al., 1988; Houghton et al., 1990.

come pregnant during the breeding season. In general, if cows calve in the spring with a BCS of 5 (where 1 = emaciated and 9 = obese), and maintain weight after calving, pregnancy rates of 80–90% will be obtained. If cows calve with BCS between 4 and 6, the effect of a one-unit change in BCS is greater than for cows that are thinner or fatter at calving.

A BCS above 4.0–5.0 (from the total range of 1–9) is vitally important for reproduction, fetal growth, lactation, and primary calf health. In addition, an ideal BCS above 5.0 is not only necessary for quality and quantity of colostrum, but also for proper lactation and subsequent rebreeding.

BCS and re-breeding

Research has shown that cows with a BCS of 4.0 or less at calving are about 50% less likely to breed back than cows with a BCS of 6.0 at calving. Also, a BCS of 4.0 before winter weather requires 28% more energy for maintenance than a cow of BCS of 6.0, because of internal fat covering that insulates the cow and maintains normal body temperature.

This affects the economics of feeding during the winter gestation period, requiring more feed to maintain or increase BCS with the intent of increasing breeding efficiency after calving.

Pre-calving weight and BCS changes also influence the interval from calving to the first estrus. It has been found that the percentage decrease in body weight from November until just prior to calving in March was correlated with the number of days to first estrus (61) and days to conception (62).

In addition, Dunn and Kaltenbach (1980) found that for each 2.2

pounds loss of body weight before calving, the percentage of cows that showed estrus by 60 days after calving decreased by 0.5%.

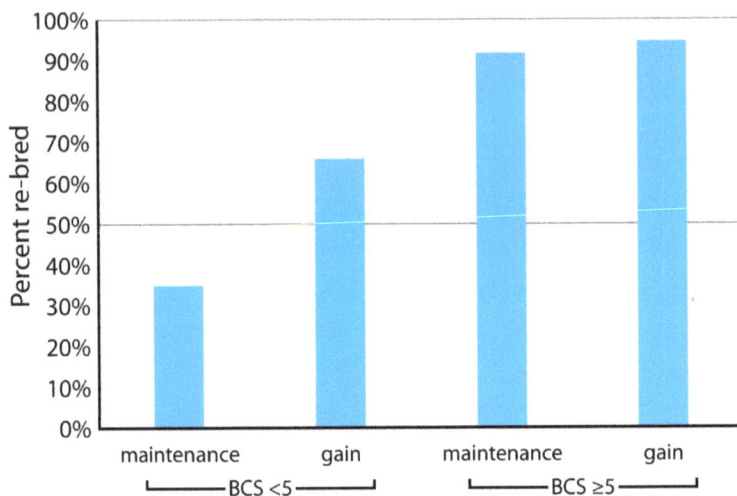

Figure 1: *Percent of heifers re-bred, by body condition score (BCS) and feeding regimen.*[3]

Body weight changes during pregnancy may also influence post-partum reproductive performance independent of BCS. Cows that were fed to maintain body weight during the last half of pregnancy had a 13% greater pregnancy rate than cows with a similar BCS at calving that had lost and regained weight.[4]

BCS and calf survival

Factors that influence the birth weight and survival of calves are many and dependent upon differences of environment, breed, genetics, nutrition, and many other determining factors. Reduced nutrient intake during the last third of pregnancy may cause reduced

3.   *Adapted from graph by Wetterman, 1993.*
4.   Selk et al., 1988.

birth weights as well as calf mortality, reduced milk production, and decreased postnatal calf growth. Past research trials have indicated that beef cows that have been fed restricted diets during late gestation have calves with lighter birth weights compared to cows with adequate nutrition. These observations have resulted in some ranchers reducing feed intake of cows, especially first calf heifers, during pregnancy in an attempt to decrease calving difficulties.

Trials in research, from multiple studies, have determined the influence of BCS and nutrient intake of mature cows during late pregnancy on fetal growth and uterine and placental development.[5] Trials that assigned cows to different feeding treatments at 180 days gestation were compared, as cows were divided into groups to achieve BCS at 260 days of gestation. At 260 days, the thin cows had a BCS of 3.7 and moderate cows had a BCS of 5.7.[6] Body weights were 922 ± 35 lb. for thin cows and 1122 ± 33 lbs. for moderate cows. Weights and lengths of the calves at slaughter were not significantly different for thin and moderate cows. The uteri were heavier in the moderate than the thin cows, but the total placental fluid volume was not altered by treatment. However, the fetal membranes and cotyledons weighed more in thin cows than in moderate cows. Increased growth of the placental membranes and cotyledons occurred in the thin cows, compared with the moderate cows, and may be the reason why calf weights were not altered at 260 days by the reduced nutrients available to the thin cows.[7] Fetal-placental changes do occur in cows during late gestation to compensate for reductions in energy intake and body energy reserves. Only major reductions in

5. Rasby et al., 1990.
6. Wetterman, 1993.
7. Wetterman, 1993.

nutrient intake result in reduced birth weight of calves.

The following table shows the correlation between BCS and uterine and placenetal tissue conditions.

Body condition	Thin	Moderate
Number of cows	8	9
Body weight	923 lbs.	1112 lbs.
Body condition score	3.7	5.7
Uterine weight	8.67 lbs.	9.67 lbs.
Placental weight	2.84 lbs.	2.34 lbs.
Cotyledonary weight	4.12 lbs.	3.17 lbs.

Table 2: Comparison of uterine and placental tissue weights of thin to moderate BCS conditions reflecting the differences in possible fetal development. Placental and fetal characteristics of cows in thin or moderate body condition on day 260 of gestation.

Recommendations related to BCS[8]

1. The body condition score (BCS) of cows at calving is the most important factor that determines if cows will become pregnant during the breeding season. To ensure good reproductive performance, spring-calving cows should calve with a BCS of 5 and heifers should have a BCS of at least 5.5.

2. Growth of the placental membranes and cotyledons is increased when nutritional intake of cows is limited during late pregnancy. It takes severe nutritional restrictions to reduce birth weights of calves from cows, but moderate nutritional restrictions will reduce the birth weight of calves from

8. Adapted from Wetterman, R.P., 1993. *Pre-calving nutrition / birth weight interaction and rebreeding efficiency.* Range Beef Cow Symposium, December 1993, Cheyenne, Wyoming

first-calf heifers.

3. Reducing the birth weights of calves from first calf heifers by nutritional restrictions does not decrease the incidence of calving difficulty, but greatly reduces postpartum reproductive performance.

It has been established that BCS at calving is the major factor that influences the percentage of cows that become pregnant during the breeding season. Nutrient intake during late gestation can influence calf birth weight, and calf birth weight is positively associated with calving difficulty.[9] Sometimes producers reduce the feed intake of first-calf heifers in an attempt to decrease birth weight of the calves and to decrease calving difficulty.

Past research has proven calving difficulty is not influenced by BCS of the heifers at calving. About one-third of the heifers in each BCS group require assistance at calving. Percentages of live calves at birth and at weaning are not influenced by BCS of the heifers at calving. [10]

Figure 1 (see earlier) shows that feeding greater amounts of energy after calving can improve the pregnancy rate or shorten the interval from calving to conception in thin heifers, but it will not compensate entirely for the poor condition of heifers at calving. In other words, increasing the plane of nutrition for heifers with BCS of 3 or 4 after calving will not allow them to rebreed as well as heifers that calve with a BCS of 5 or greater.

Results also indicate there is no advantage, as far as reproduction is concerned, to feeding greater amounts of energy to heifers after calving if they calve in good body condition, since only about 53% of the

9. Bellows et al., 1971

10. Wetterman, 1993.

heifers that calved in good body condition and gained weight were pregnant by 90 days postpartum.

It is a recommended practice to plan to have heifers calve earlier than the cow herd, so that they will breed back and calve at similar times the next year.[11] First calf-heifers need 2-4 weeks more time to adjust to lactation, clear up uterine discharges, gain body weight, and return to estrus.

Calving

Dr. Mark Hilton's Calving Tips[12]

1. Calve in a clean, dry environment. "Clean" means a place where you didn't winter cows. Moisture is particularly important as moisture can be a calf-killer, so calve on well-drained land.

2. The solution to pollution is often dilution: ideally, calves should be born outside, on pasture where animals are *spread out*. Of course, ambient temperature is a factor, too, but being outside in weather conducive to calving remains best.

3. Keep the herd *out* of the barn. If cows and calves have access to a barn, it can become an incubator for serious infection and disease. Letting calves into a well-bedded shelter during inclement weather is fine, but keep the cows out of the barn.

4. With beef cows, we don't always know whether the calves have nursed, or how much. If you're unsure whether a calf

---

11. Wetterman, 1993.
12. Taken from *Beef* magazine, October 2009. W. Mark Hilton, DVM, is a clinical associate professor of beef production medicine at Purdue University Veterinary School in West Lafayette, IN.

has nursed (calf seems clueless, cow's udder is tight, or the calf appears gaunt), milk out the cow and get 2-3 quarts. Tube-feed or suckle the calf with colostrum or a quality colostrum supplement as soon as possible. (After day one, use a combination of milk and electrolytes.) *It's critical that this is done within 12 hours of birth.*

5. Now, to see if the calf does know how to nurse, pen the calf away from the cow but allow nose-to-nose contact. A short gate in the corner of a pen works best. In 6-8 hours, put the calf with its dam and see if he nurses. If the calf does nurse, you're in good shape for minimizing problems. If not, you'll have to tube the calf twice daily until the calf figures it out. Using a black-colored lambs nipple (on a glass pop bottle) usually works much better than the large red ones that come with the plastic quart bottles.

6. If the calf is slow to learn to nurse, *don't force the calf* to suckle twice per day; you'll get frustrated and so will the calf. Instead, try about once every other day, and see if the calf is getting any smarter. Be sure to castrate that calf; and, if you get many similar calves, send the sire to market and buy a bull that will increase vigor at birth.

7. Increasing calf vigor at birth helps ensure adequate colostrum intake. If this is a concern, improving hybrid vigor with crossbreeding should help. The use of injectable vitamin B complexes with fortified vitamin B 12 will stimulate the calf's appetite reflex.

8. Keep cows separate from first-calf heifers. Because cows have been exposed to more pathogens than heifers, the calves from older cows should gain more immunity after nursing their colostrum. When calves are exposed to a disease agent,

the calves from the heifers will likely get sick while the calves from cows may not. The bad news, though, is that once the sick calves contaminate the environment, even the healthy calves may get sick.

9. *Don't pay good money for disease.* Calving season isn't the time to introduce new animals into the herd. Don't buy new cows with calves, and never buy a calf for a cow that lost hers. In fact, all new purchases should be quarantined from your herd for 30-60 days.

10. Vaccinate if necessary. Some calf diseases are diminished by using vaccine on the dam or on the calf itself. *Check with your herd-health veterinarian* for recommendations for your geographic area.

11. Move the herd? Learn how to adopt the Sandhills Calving System to your herd. Yes, this works best if you have sandy ground, but the concept of moving yet-to-calve cows to a new area works everywhere. Work with your herd-health veterinarian to see how it can be used on your farm or ranch.

Moving cows without calves is easier than moving pairs, and labor can be managed to accommodate cow movement a week in advance. Information from pregnancy testing will provide help in managing cow movements (early and later calving groups), as cows expected to calve later can be fed in another area, minimizing crowding and manure contamination that may increase risks of coccidian outbreaks.

The main advantage is that keeping older calves with their dams eliminates the problem of older calves passing microorganisms to younger ones. Cows that have not calved can be moved to a new, clean area for those younger calves to be born later away from older calves, preventing risk of infection.

Sandhills Calving Rotational Management

Pasture 8 (empty)	Pasture 7 (empty)	Pasture 6 (empty)	Pasture 5 (empty)
Pasture 1 3-4 week old pairs	**Pasture 2** 2-week-old pairs	**Pasture 3** 1-week-old pairs	**Pasture 4** calving

Table 3. The Sandhills Calving System: During the fifth week, cows that are calving are in pasture 4, with pairs in the first three pastures.

The use of the Nebraska Sandhills System of calving is fundamentally sound, as the cows that have not calved in 10-14 days are moved to a new area to prevent the older calves from infecting the new-born calves.

Grouping cows

Although grouping cattle together at calving in small areas allows for efficient watching and reduces problems with dystocia (obstructed labour), this practice also increases disease problems by six-fold or more.[13] A rancher has a significant decision to make in grouping cows to minimize dystocia problems, or by not grouping, avoid the risk of increased calf sickness due to diarrhea and other infectious diseases that occur during the first three weeks of life.

Timing of Calving

Recent data collected form USADA NAHMS (2008) show a marked difference in mortality of calves born in the first three weeks of the calving period (see the chart below), compared to those calves born later in the calving period. Improvements in animal health technology and progress made in beef cattle management have

---

13. Hilton, 2006.

helped increase beef production dramatically in the past fifty years, yet calf health remains a challenging problem, and mortality from diarrheas and respiratory disease remain significant factors impacting economic success.

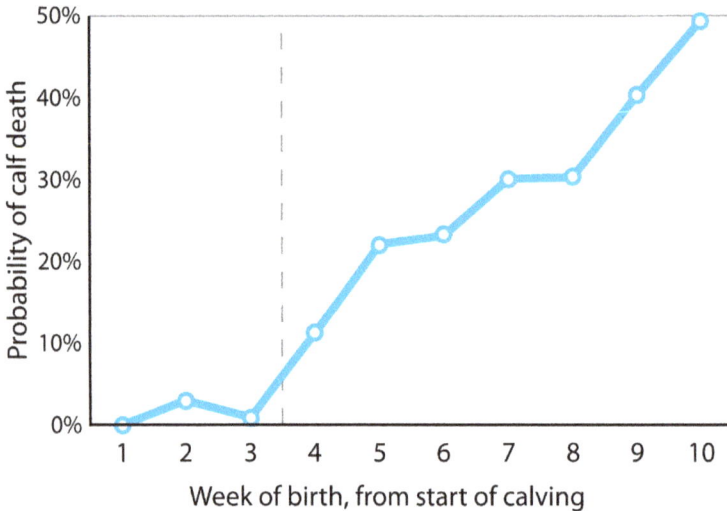

Figure 2: *Probability of calf death, related to time of birth in calving period. Calves born in the first three weeks have higher survival ability than those born later in the calving cycle.*[14]

This figure shows the dramatic increase in mortality for calves born after three weeks from the start of calving. Calves born after eight weeks from the start of calving have a *ten times higher* incidence of mortality, emphasizing the importance of "tight breeding dates" and the importance of having two thirds of calves born in the first three weeks of the calving period. The latter goal is compatible with the fact that most cows will be rebred during the next breeding season, as the post-partum period is longer for necessary uterine involution and timely estrous to begin for breeding.

14. *Data obtained from White, 2011. Original source of Smith, 2003.*

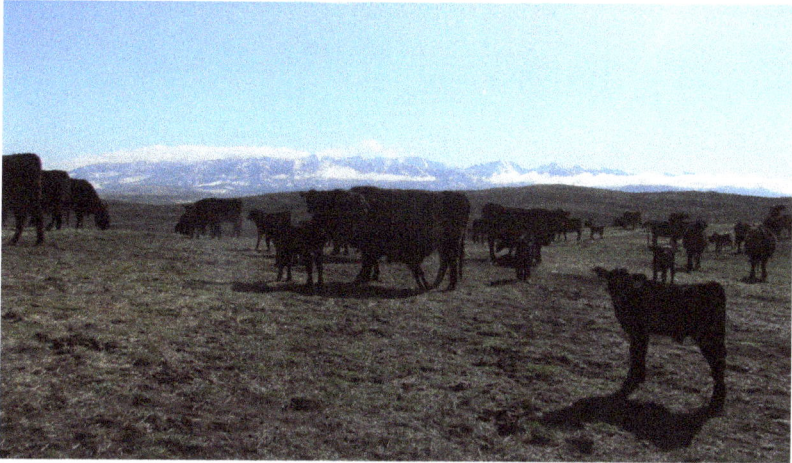

2

Newborn Calf Health

The first three weeks are a critical period in determining calf survival and economic success.

The chart on the following page shows that the percentage of un-weaned calf death is 31.3% in the first 24 hours after birth, and furthermore, that two-thirds of all deaths of un-weaned calves occur before three weeks of age.

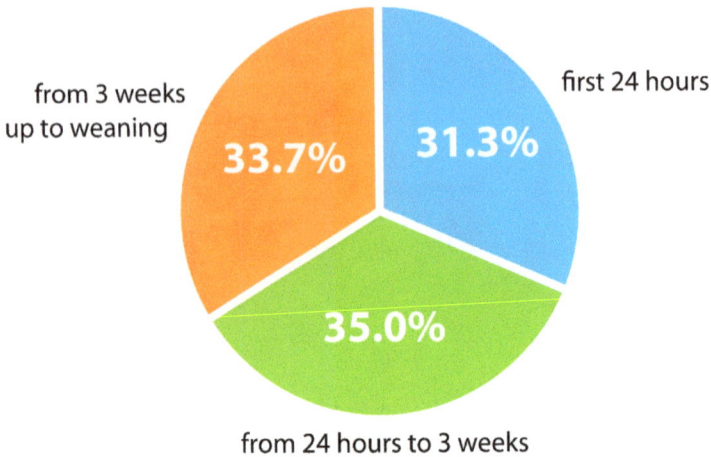

from 3 weeks up to weaning — 33.7%

first 24 hours — 31.3%

35.0%

from 24 hours to 3 weeks

Figure 3: Calf deaths, by age at death, for operations in which any unweaned calves died or were lost from all causes in 2007.[15]

Ranchers that increase their labor and attention to calves during the first three weeks of life have higher weaned percentages than those who do not increase attention or labor during this period.[16] By increasing attention to calf health during this period, morbidity and mortality will decrease, resulting in economic success at weaning time.

Keys to newborn calf survival

The newborn calf's ability to respond to disease is determined by these factors:

- Mostly critically, the protection given by immunoglobulins from colostrum the calf has consumed, especially in the first 12 hours; as well as

---

15. *Adapted from figure provided by USDA-NAHMS, 2007.*

16. USDA-NAHMS, 2007.

+ additional stress on the calf during the disease challenge,

+ the ability to meet energy needs,

+ severity of the infection and the organism causing the infection problem.

Many ranchers do not understand that the calf's energy needs during the first few hours of life can deeply affect health. New physiological processes in the calf's body are initiated by directing energy to them. Add stress from cold, wetness, or wind, and energy can be lost in minutes. Increased energy is required to compensate for these environmental stressors.

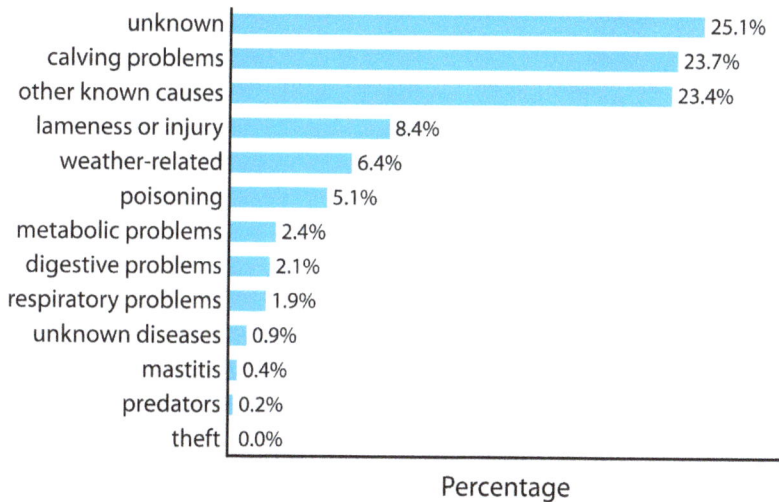

Cause	Percentage
unknown	25.1%
calving problems	23.7%
other known causes	23.4%
lameness or injury	8.4%
weather-related	6.4%
poisoning	5.1%
metabolic problems	2.4%
digestive problems	2.1%
respiratory problems	1.9%
unknown diseases	0.9%
mastitis	0.4%
predators	0.2%
theft	0.0%

Percentage

Figure 4: *Primary causes of calf death during the first 6 months of life.*[17]

An understanding of management factors that influence infection and disease is critical for decreasing mortality and increasing calf viability and health. Understanding this concept and making correc-

17. *Adapted from figure provided by USDA-NAHMS, 2008.*

tions is a key factor in success the first week of the calf's life.

Many times, the unknown causes shown in the graph above are un-detected pneumonia and dehydration problems not observed before mortality. In the Northern Great Plains, pneumonia-related diseases are a primary concern in causing unknown mortality in beef calves during the spring calving season.

Recommendation: After the second calf lost to an unknown cause of death, consider necropsying the second calf to identify the diagnosis or cause of death. Necropsies can produce valuable knowledge of infectious diseases, and liver biopsies can also be obtained at this time to evaluate the current mineral program on your ranch.

The necropsy section of this book details the correct methods needed to identify pathological causes and trauma-induced mortality.

Colostrum

Considering the total health requirements of beef cattle, *there is no more important factor than colostrum nutrition and intake during the first three-to-four hours after birth.*

Compared to mature bovine milk, colostrum contains higher total solids (27.6% vs. 12.3%), higher protein (14.9% vs. 2.8%), and slightly higher fat (6.7% vs. 4.4%).

Colostrum quality and quantity are not only vital to survival ability, but can also affect feedlot performance, even one year after intake, and are important health factors throughout life.

The importance of colostrum has been noted for centuries, but until recently we did not understand the complexity and importance of colostrum's influence on life-time health. The nutrients necessary for production of specific colostrum components are just now being identified. Recent research has discovered the relationship between timely and adequate colostrum consumption and the economics of gain and performance in the feedlot, up to one year after nursing at birth. We now understand that quality colostrum consumed by the calf during the first few hours is one of the most important production requirements necessary for maximal performance and reproduction later in life.

This concept, which can't be overstressed, is the most important factor toward calf health and beef calf production during the first months of life. It is directly related to economic return.

Cowboy message: Colostrum = $$$$.

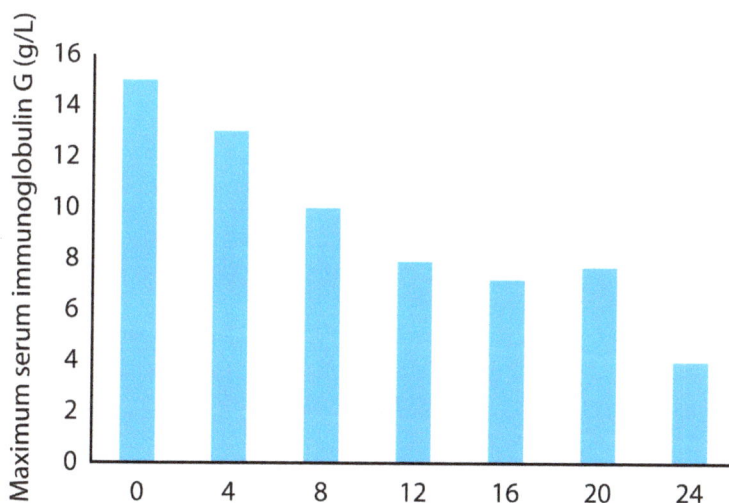

Figure 5: *Immunoglobulin levels, by age at first feeding. A 50% drop in the first 12 hours.*[18]

18. Data are a composite of various reports in the literature.

Declining absorption

The most successful producers are those that make sure adequate amounts of colostrum are suckled during the first 3-4 hours. The ability to absorb colostrum (large fat molecules) decreases markedly after birth as the cellular structure in the intestine changes and the large molecules cannot be absorbed. The "time clock" starts when the *first fluid is ingested* by the calf. This is very important when considering the window of opportunity for colostrum absorption.

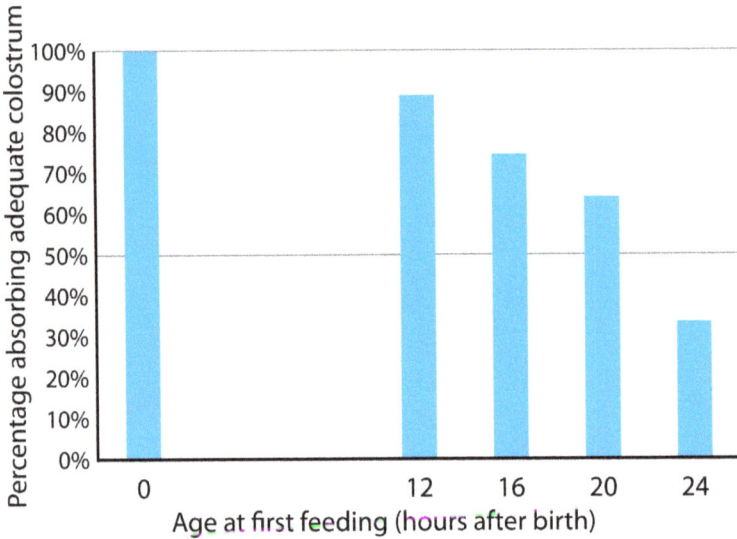

Figure 6: *Percentage of calves absorbing adequate colostrum, by age at first feeding. Note the difference between this chart and Figure 5 (which shows the quantity of immunoglobulins absorbed).*

Even when calves are given adequate amounts of colostrum 12 hours after birth, the percentage of colostrum absorbed is much lower than when given in the first few hours, supporting the "time concept" of nursing colostrum. Calves that do not receive an adequate amount of colostrum in a timely manner have increased morbidity and mortality numbers during the first months of life.[19]

By minimizing stress and ensuring adequate colostrum intake, success can be achieved in the first few days after birth, and this carries throughout the entire life of the calf. Data indicate increased weaning weights, increased feed utilization, and increased reproductive performance in heifer calves that had adequate or increased levels of colostrum during the first 3-4 hours after birth.

Colostrum and immunity

A calf is born with a naïve immune system. Calves, unlike other mammals, have placental tissue that does not allow immunoglobulins (pre-formed antibodies) to pass through the maternal blood to the fetus.

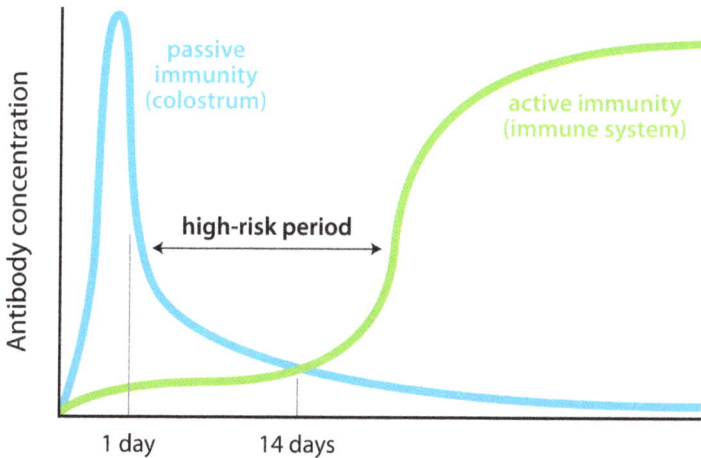

Figure 7: *Representation of passive immunity (from colostrum) versus the calf's adaptive and innate immune response, related to time after birth.*[20]

19. AM J Vet Res 56: 1149

20. Composite of various reports in the literature.

However, colostrum provides 80% of the immunoglobulins necessary for life. Therefore, the need for passive immune protection through colostrum intake is *greater in calves* than with other species of livestock.

Figure 7 (previous page) shows how the calf is almost completely dependent on colostrum for immunity during the first week of life. The calf's immune system is vast and complex, is slow to develop, and requires energy intake to respond effectively. A calf's immune system does not begin to develop significantly until after two weeks of life, and it is believed that full development does not occur until at least 8 months of age (weaning time).

The risk period from one to two weeks after birth is when passive immunity from colostrum begins to drop, but the calf's own immune system has not yet developed to meet infection challenges. This is the period when major clinical infections dominate, such as diarrheas and pneumonias. This explains why mortality is higher during this period (as shown at the start of this chapter).

In addition to providing immunoglobulins for immunity, colostrum is also rich in lactoferrin, a protein that prevents bacterial multiplication and helps bind iron that is necessary for bacterial growth. Immunoglobulins themselves are also an important source of energy and vitamins.

Colostrum and vaccination

One of the most misunderstood aspects of colostrum is its influence on vaccination. Many producers believe that the antibodies within colostrum block the calf's response to any attempted vaccinations. In fact, the calf's own lack of immune development during the first two weeks is the reason that most vaccine products do not result in antibody production early in life.

Although measuring antibody response after the calf is vaccinated yields a zero response in titer levels, recent discoveries indicate that other immunological advantages are obtained by vaccinating calves, responses that cannot be measured by titer response. The first of these is an excellent B-cell memory response that shows up later (which helps in the booster effect). B-cells are the precursors of plasma cells responsible for antibody production. Many producers use early (day 1-5) vaccinations because of the effect on B-cell memory that improve response to vaccinations at branding time.

Also, cell-mediated response (at the point of infection) is increased by early vaccination, even when paired with high levels of colostrum, and especially with attenuated vaccines.

Cows vaccinated prior to calving with commercially available killed-scour products have shown very positive responses in the form of increased antibody levels in colostrum at calving. Economic advantages have been shown with using scour vaccine products in almost all herds. Costs incurred compared to increased calf health alone have been very positive.

Losses from scours is still the number one health problem in many areas, and losses from one day of scour sickness can amount to *over $30.00 of weight loss and decreased performance after weaning, even if treatment is successful after one day.* Calves that are sick for more than one day usually require treatment. *They end up as much as fifty pounds lighter at weaning, with permanent intestinal problems that decrease nutrient absorption later in life.*

Many times, microscopic tissue changes resulting from pathogen damage to intestinal villa are permanent. They affect performance later in the feedlot in the form of decreased feed efficiency and carcass grade and quality. Modified live viral (MLV) vaccines for respiratory disease prevention have shown similar results and gains. Results from killed or inactivated respiratory viral vaccines have been less effective and not as promising.[21]

Colostrum, weaning weight, and economic impact

Immunoglobulin levels	Inadequate	Adequate
Number of calves	60	183
Morbidity	25.0%	4.9%
Mean weight at weaning	471 lbs.	495 lbs.

Table 4: Level of colostrum intake compared to calf morbidity and final weaning weight.[22]

The preceding table shows a sizable increase in weaning weights of calves receiving adequate levels of colostrum.

Morbidity levels are increased by more than 5 times in calves that receive inadequate colostrum during the first 6 months, compared to those calves receiving adequate colostrum. Performance as yearlings is reduced in terms of average daily gain, increased morbidity, and even in carcass traits, which all affect profit. Much attention is directed to increased health with vaccinations, anti-parasites, and growth implants, yet none of these are as important as making sure the calf has adequate colostrum at birth.

In a herd of 100 cows, the difference in economic gain on weaning weights alone amounts to $3420.00 (24 lbs × 95 surviving calves

21. Smith, 2009.

22. Slide courtesy of Dr. Brad White, Kansas State University (2011; adapted from smith, 2005). [Am j. Vet. Res. 56: 1149]

x $1.50 /lb.). This is without considering the economic gain from the improved morbidity rate, which reduces health costs (treatment, labor, drugs) and eliminates the 2% mortality loss, providing an additional $2800.00 of economic gain.[23]

Altogether, the total economic loss caused by inadequate colostrum intake *approaches $7000 for a 100-cow herd.* This is a huge amount when considering the total profit in a typical year in a 100-cow herd. For this reason, proper pre-calving nutrition and colostrum management provide an excellent return value compared to input costs.

Plasma protein level at 24 hrs.	Total gain
Adequate	570 lbs.
Inadequate	548 lbs.

Table 5: *This table demonstrates the overall impact of colostrum intake on total gain. (Gain is for a 125–140 day feeding period in the feedlot, with the same intake of feed for both groups.) Inadequate colostrum causes intermediate factors, such as higher incidence of respiratory infection, which in turn affect the lifetime health of the calf and reduce its total gain.*[24]

Studies also show that calves with inadequate colostrum intake have 3-9 times the morbidity than calves with adequate intake, and over 5 times the mortality.[25] This often results in six times more pneumonia and ten times more enteritis (scours) in calves that do not receive adequate colostrum during the first 3-4 hours after birth.[26]

---

23. Sager, 2011.

24. Chart taken from Smith, 2003. [Am. J. Vet. Res. 56: 1149]

25. Hilton, 2005.

26. Sager, 2015.

Immunoglobulin levels	Inadequate	Adequate
Difference in morbidity	+510%	=
Difference in weaning weight	=	+24 lbs.

Table 6: Serum IgG levels at 24 hours and calf health and gain from first 8 months to weaning.

The morbidity in calves that receive inadequate levels of colostrum is over five times the morbidity in calves that receive adequate levels of colostrum. This difference is reflected in increased health costs in treatment, labor, and a difference in weaning weights of 24 pounds.

Colostrum and treatment outcomes

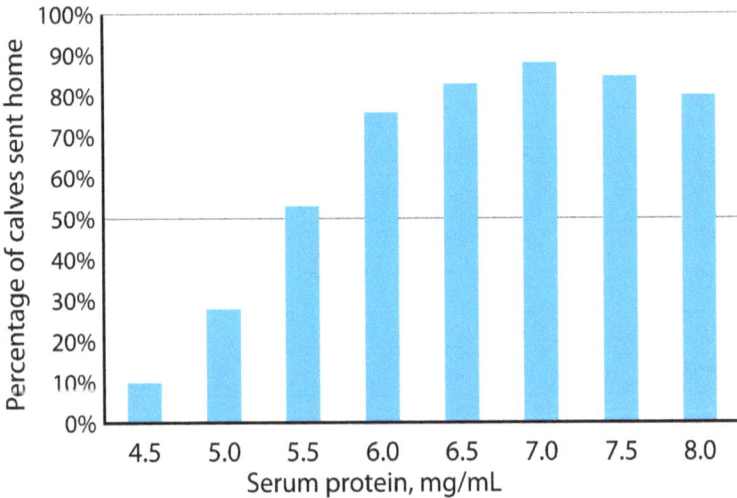

Figure 8: Success of intensive IV treatment, by serum protein level. [27]

This data was prepared from records of over 3000 calves treated for either scours or scours with pneumonia, over a 35-year career. The data shows that serum protein levels above 6.0 mg/mL resulted in

27. Bob Sager, DVM, from period 1975-2010.

a higher percentage of success in IV treatment, because of adequate colostrum intake. Colostrum intake was important in providing passive immunity that improved treatment success and increased the percentage of calves sent home. Calves were evaluated for serum protein levels when IV catheters were placed, and a refractometer evaluation was completed before the client left for home to give a prognosis based on data information from past years' data. This provided information to clients to determine whether the client should continue treatment and gave a basis for success in treatment.

Other properties of colostrum

Ingestion of colostrum produces bowel movement by natural laxatives, causing passage of the meconium.[28]

The Importance of Feeding Schedule to Calf Survival

Calves should nurse in the first 30-45 minutes after birth. They should then nurse several times during the first 6 hours of life, so that they receive 2 quarts of quality colostrum in the first 6 hours, and 4 quarts over the first 12 hours. Calf success and survival is highly dependent on this benchmark.

Total fluid intake the first 24 hours should be between 10–15% of the total body weight of the calf. A rough guide is 1 pint per 10–12 lbs. over each 24-hour period, for the first few days.

28. Radostits, 2007.

Figure 9 (below) shows the large drop in absorption of colostrum between birth and 9 hours, due to the physiological closure of the epithelial cells in the intestinal tissues, which prevents large nutrient molecules (colostrum) from being transported across the epithelial cell surfaces for tissue absorption and metabolism.

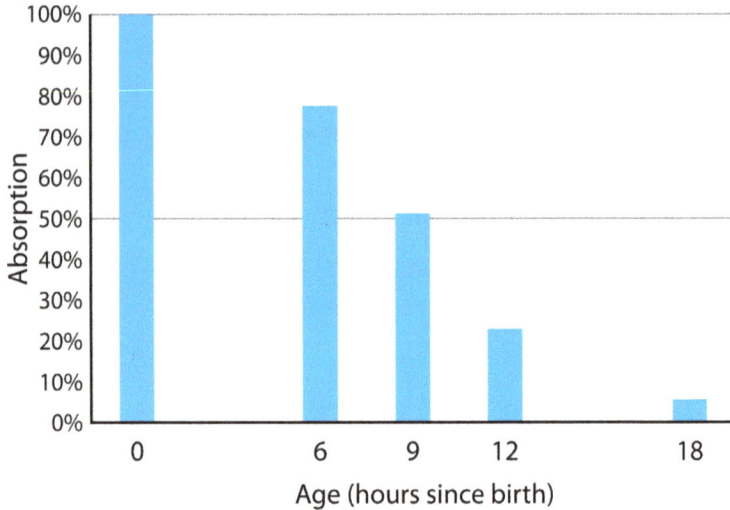

Figure 9: *Percent of immunoglobulin absorbed, by age in hours since birth.*[29]

Figure 10 (opposite page) reflects the importance of multiple feedings of colostrum, however, the time factor is critical for total absorption, and is more critical than total amount consumed. Thus, it is necessary to feed colostrum multiple times in the first 4-8 hours for maximum immunoglobulin absorption and passive protection. The use of multiple feedings at an early age (4-8 hours) has an effect in both percent absorbed and total amount absorbed, as a higher percent of any volume is absorbed when given at an earlier age.

29. From Jacobsen, K. L *Colostrum Management* at http://www.FarmLLC.org/ custom3.html

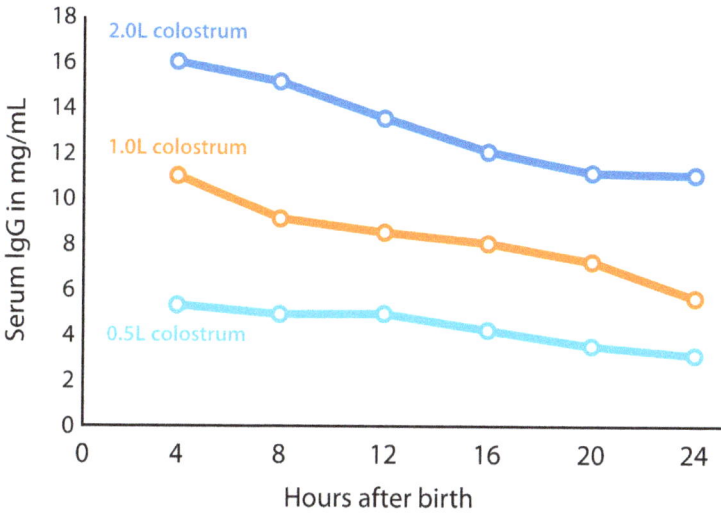

Figure 10: *Serum immunoglobulins by age and by amount of colostrum fed.*[30]

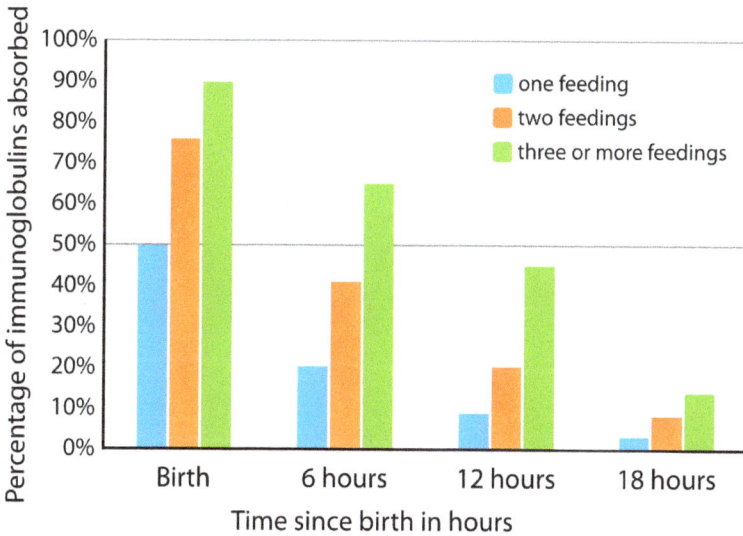

Figure 11: *Total amount of immunoglobulins absorbed, by number of feedings and hours since birth. (Data from several sources).*

30. Data adapted from a chart from Merrick's website.

Figure 11 (previous page) shows increased total immunoglobulins absorbed with increased feedings of colostrum, but also shows the influence of time after birth when feedings occur. With increased time after birth, increased feedings do not increase the amounts of immunoglobulins absorbed because of partial closure of epithelial tissues in the intestinal tract. This data also shows the importance of multiple feedings in increasing total immunoglobulins absorbed.

Table 7 below shows increased total immunoglobulins absorbed with increased feedings of colostrum, but also shows the influence of time after birth when feedings occur. With increased time after birth, increased feedings do not increase the amounts of immuno-globulins absorbed because of partial closure of epithelial tissues in the intestinal tract. This data also shows the importance of multiple feedings in increasing total immunoglobulins absorbed.

Colostrum intake	Number of herds	Mortality (7-180 days)
2–4 lbs.	18	15.3%
5–8 lbs.	16	9.9%
8–10 lbs.	26	6.5%

Table 7: Colostrum intake versus calf mortality after one week of age. Mortality percentage represents the average of the mortality rates of individual herds.

The table above shows the importance of increased amounts of colostrum in decreasing the mortality in calves after one week of age. By increasing the amount of colostrum threefold (from 2–4 to 8–10 lbs.), the mortality drops by nearly two thirds (from 15.3% to 6.5%).

Table 8 (opposite page) shows that the concentration of antibody content in the first milking is higher than in later milkings.

	1st milking (colostrum)	11th milking (whole milk)
Total solids	23.0%	13.0%
Total protein	4.8%	2.5%
Casein	4.8%	2.5%
Immunoglobulins	6.0%	0.1%
Fat	6.7%	4.0%
Lactose	2.7%	4.9%
Minerals	1.0%	0.7%
Specific gravity	1.056	1.032

Table 8: Colostrum Quality and Absorption in Baby Calves. Approximate composition of colostrum and whole milk.[31]

Note the difference of concentration of antibodies or immunoglobulins in the first milking verses the 11th milking in the same cow—a difference of 66 times the concentration in the first to 11th milking.

Supplementation

Pre-calving nutrition is essential for producing quality colostrum. However, even in well-managed herds, *it is common for approximately one third of the first calving heifers to have marginal colostrum quality and quantity.*

Therefore, there is often a need to supplement colostrum intake with additional natural colostrum, or with available commercial colostrum-supplement products.

31. Table and values courtesy of Duane N. Rice, extension veterinarian and Douglas G. Rogers, diagnostic pathologist of the University of Minnesota.

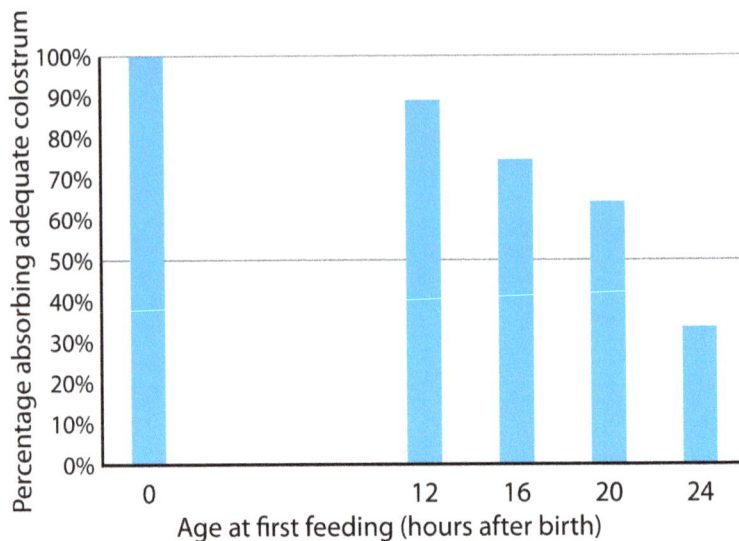

Figure 6 (repeated): *Percentage of calves absorbing adequate colostrum, by age at first feeding.*[32]

Detecting inadequate colostrum intake

In certain situations, calves will display reoccurring infections due to reduction of normal immune function. During the first few weeks of life, this can occur due to inadequate colostrum intake. The symptoms could be any of the following:[33]

+ Repeated infections during the first 6 weeks of life

+ Low white blood cell (WBC) levels

+ Unusual disease problems that have not occurred before with "normal" calves

+ Infections that respond poorly to antibiotics or treatment

32. Merrick's handout, 2011.

33. Sager, 2000.

The signs above may indicate inadequate colostrum intake, but there may also be other causes that have reduced the calf's immune function, such as:

+ Use of modified live virus (MLV) vaccines at an early age, compromising a less-mature immune system

+ Poor energy intake

+ Use of corticosteroids (for anti-inflammatory purposes), causing a depressed immune system by decreasing circulating white blood cells and decreasing innate immune system function

Testing whether a calf has received adequate colostrum intake can be done easily *by testing for the total protein in the calf's blood by using a refractometer* (ask your vet). Total protein levels should be above 5.0–5.5, or equal to over 1000 mg/dl of IgG in the blood serum.

When in doubt, tube with colostrum (it can almost never be too much). Fifteen minutes of colostrum in the first few hours can save a calf.

Freezing colostrum

Freeze extra colostrum from healthy vaccinated middle-aged cows from the herd for use later. Cows may be milked out completely after they calve. Remove at least some extra colostrum from older cows that have produced good quality colostrum.

Colostrum, when properly frozen and thawed, remains good almost indefinitely. Save this extra colostrum for calves from other cows that produce abnormal colostrum (mastitis, bloody or watery colostrum). Freeze colostrum in containers of approximately 3–4 pints (1.5–2L or Qt) for storage and thawing.

Freezing colostrum in this way is good preparation for future needs, because each container holds an appropriate amount for a single feeding. Before frozen colostrum is needed, remove it from the freezer and let it slowly thaw to room temperature.

Important: Do not heat colostrum to high temperatures (above 125°F). High temperatures denature the protein components of colostrum, destroying the immunoglobulin value.

Important: Do not use a microwave to thaw colostrum. Microwaves can heat unevenly or too quickly, denaturing the protein.

Commercial colostrum supplements

Commercial colostrum products are available and are proven to supplement normal colostrum. These should be used with warm water as directed and fed as soon as a problem in nursing is confirmed. Emphasize timely and frequent doses of colostrum, given in a careful and sanitary manner.

Commercial supplements are popular because of convenience, as it takes time to bring a heifer or cow in, milk out colostrum, and then tube or suckle a calf. A tubing of supplemental commercial colostrum will benefit the calf in a timely manner.

Natural colostrum is higher in total immunoglobulins, thus of more value to the calf, but several treatments of commercial products are better than waiting for a chilled calf to rise and suckle the cow. Approximate costs are around $9.00-12.00 per bag, each of which will make 4 liters of supplement. A recommended volume is 1-2 liters per feeding. Considering time and convenience this is an excellent value.

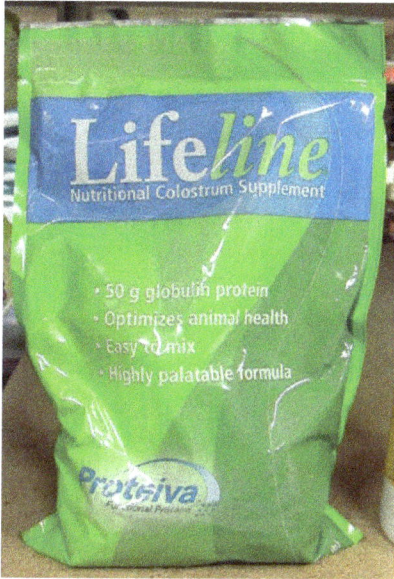

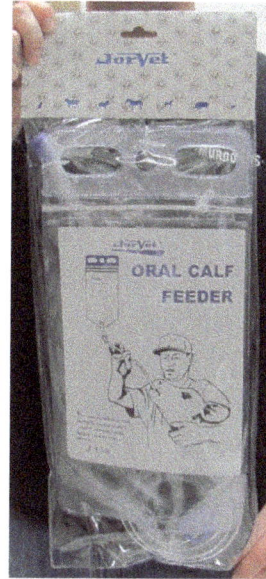

Image P01 (left): A commercial colostrum supplement. Used for drenching or suckling the calf after birth. Several commercial formulations exist. These can be very helpful with convenience and timing, which are the most important considerations.

Image P02 (right): Calf feeder bag used to drench the calf with electrolytes, fluids, or colostrum supplement. These can be carried on horseback or in a 4-wheeler, with warm water in a thermos or plastic cooler for convenience.

Cowboy tip: Commercial colostrum produces net profit at weaning time compared to no colostrum. It is a value-adding product with significant results.

Septicemia

Septicemia is a serious complication that can result from infections that occur at birth or immediately after birth.

If a microorganism or its toxins gain entry to the calf's circulating blood, this causes a mass "shotgun" spread of the microorganisms or toxins into every tissue and organ within minutes. The most susceptible and most severely affected organs are the filtering organs: kidneys, liver, and lung tissues. This overwhelms the newborn calf's ability to respond, resulting in a high rate of death.

Septicemia in calves is usually the result of a bacterial infection that occurs at birth or immediately after birth. The route of infection can be the blood of a sick dam, an infected placenta, the calf's umbilical cord, the mouth, the nose (inhalation) or a wound.

Most infections enter through the calf's umbilical area. Iodine solution to this area will dramatically decrease the incidence of septicemia.

A secondary source of infection is from other calves during the first few weeks of life.

Septicemia is the most severe problem that a calf can develop early in life. Infections are life-threatening, cost of treatment is high, and the survival rate is low.

Detecting septicemia

The early signs of septicemia are subtle, but include the following:

+ The calf is usually depressed, weak, and reluctant to stand. It may suckle poorly within the first 5 days after birth. Of these signs, depression is the most pronounced.

+ The calf may develop swollen joints, meningitis, cloudy eyes, and/or a large, tender navel.

+ The calf may develop diarrhea or pneumonia. Septicemia

can also be caused by diarrhea-causing organisms.

+ The calf will not necessarily have a fever. Many septic calves have normal or even below-normal temperatures.

+ Most septic calves have a history of inadequate colostrum intake.

Treating septicemia

These are severe infections that require immediate intensive treatment, usually requiring IV fluids, antibiotics, and intensive care and treatment for success. Success is dependent on removing infected umbilical tissues, supportive fluid therapy to flush infection and toxins from the body tissues, and supportive care as the calf is usually too sick to nurse. Septicemia is life-threatening and often results in unsuccessful treatment outcomes, even with intensive treatment.

Summary and Cowboy Tips

+ Pre-calving nutrition is very important for producing quality colostrum.

+ Make sure the calf nurses in the first 30–45 minutes of life. The ability to absorb colostrum drops dramatically after birth.

+ When in doubt, tube colostrum in the first 3–4 hours, and again 2–3 hours later.

+ It is common (even in well-managed herds) for approximately one third of the first calving heifers to have marginal colostrum quality and quantity. Be aware of the signs of inadequate intake and be prepared to supplement.

+ Prefer frozen natural colostrum to commercial products,

as it contains higher levels of natural immunoglobulins.

+ However, use commercial colostrum products as needed for ease and convenience, or when natural colostrum is unavailable.

+ Remember that two thirds of all calf deaths occur in the first 96 hours.[34]

+ Remember that colostrum is vital not only to survival, but also to feedlot performance (even one year after intake) and is an important health factor throughout life.

---

34. USDA-NAHMS, 2007, and Smith, 2009,

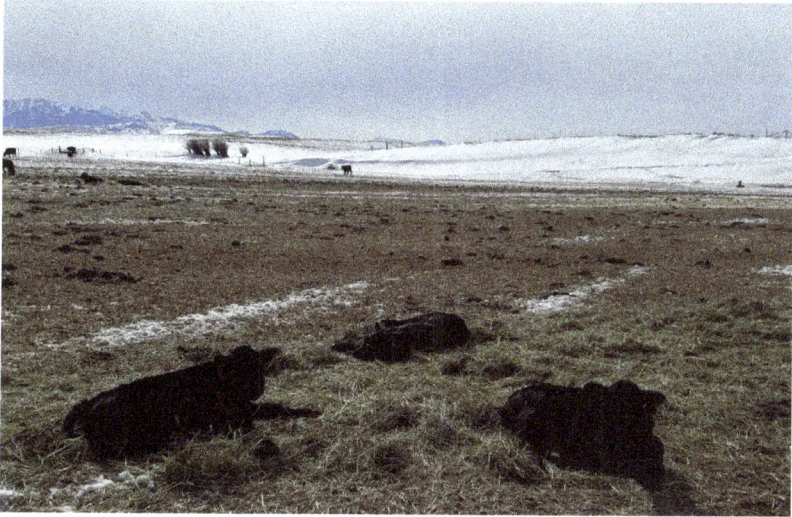

3

Diarrhea (Scours)

After deaths related to dystocia (difficulties in pregnancy or calving), which represent more than 30% of calf deaths, the next most common problem is diarrhea (13–14%). Because of the use of low-birth-weight bulls with shorter gestation times, the prevalence of dystocia has dramatically dropped in recent years, so diarrhea now represents a larger percentage of post-calving problems.

Beef cattle producers indicate that infectious diarrhea in newborn calves accounts for over 20% of the economic impact in their production, and accounts for more than 50% of the deaths.[35] Diarrhea is still the most important cause of sickness and death of beef calves.[36]

Some herds experience 10–25% of the calves with some degree of diarrhea incidence, with death loss sometimes exceeding 5%.[37] In recent years, excellent control has been achieved with the use of popular scour vaccination programs. However, the incidence of protozoan infections (coccidia and cryptosporidia) is now causing concern in herds that have experienced bacterial scours in the past. (Calving on the same ground each year increases this problem.)

An overview of diarrhea-causing diseases

Diarrhea-causing diseases are usually grouped into three classes: bacterial, viral, and other (including parasites). The most common cause of diarrhea is bacterial.

Death from diarrhea is usually due to dehydration, loss of electrolytes, and body differences in body chemistry (including acid-base balance). The infectious agent that causes diarrhea can be from many different sources, but the *dehydration and electrolyte loss are what kill, and are the most important factors in death loss versus success.*

In addition, many diarrhea-causing organisms excrete a highly potent toxin that destroys epithelial (gut) tissue, causing permanent damage which reduces future health and economic performance. The toxin can also cause ulcers and is damaging to internal organs if absorbed. It is also very neurotoxic, causing depression along with

35. Radostits et al., 2007.

36. Smith, 2003.

37. Sager, 2000.

loss of appetite and movement, often reflecting in secondary pneumonias.

Dehydration and acidosis are life-threatening and should be treated first. Treatment should also focus on eliminating the organism from the intestinal tract, and on controlling the diarrhea itself (the body's attempted method of removing the organism).

Treatment with antibiotics should only be done if recommended by professionals, as these organisms have strong resistance. Not only does this make antibiotics less effective, use of antibiotics will also destroy "good" organisms that would normally help to minimize infection. (As an exception, Amoxicillin trihydrate has been one of the few antibiotics that has resulted in success for E. coli infections.)

When diarrhea problems occur

One common characteristic of diarrhea-causing diseases is attachment to the gut lining (epithelial mucosa). This attachment allows these organisms to populate the local gut areas, instead of being passed as other organisms are. This factor is age-dependent, which is why calves of two weeks and older do not experience as many incidents of diarrhea, and the incidents are not as severe.

Most problems with diarrhea occur within the first three weeks of birth.[38]

Figure 12 (next page) shows that more than 95% of the deaths attributed to scours occur between days 7–21 (from the end of the first week through week three).

---

38. Sager, 2000.

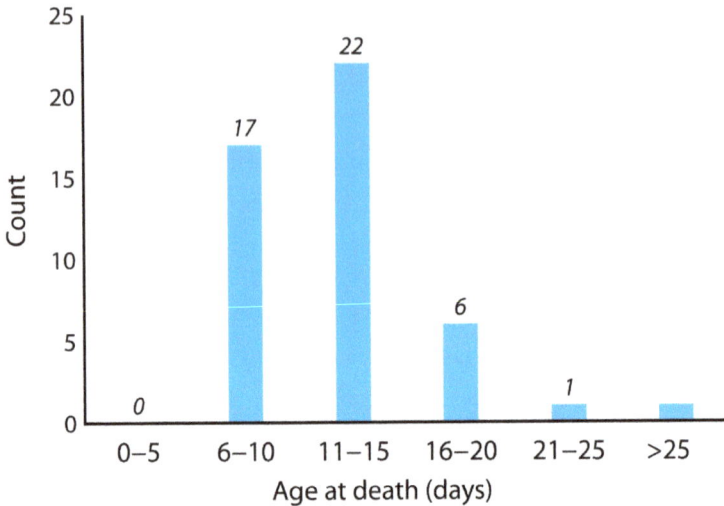

Figure 12: *Age of calves at death, for deaths attributable to scours. Most calves died between 6 and 15 days of age.*[39]

Diarrhea: a cowboy diagnosis

Table 9 (facing page) provides some simple guidelines for determining which organism may be causing diarrhea in a calf. This chart is a guideline only. Days of incidence will vary, and color and consistency of diarrhea will vary with incidence and infection rates.

It is rare for a calf to have bacterial scours after day 22, so scours after that day should be examined for coccidia, Clostridium spp., or cryptosporidia, and a fecal sample should be examined microscopically or sent for diagnosis evaluation.

Samples can be easily checked under a microscope with a specific proper stain. This can be completed at the local veterinary office, as most human clinics will not accept veterinary samples because

39. Data from *Sandhills Calving System*, Smith, 2003.

of bio-security measures in place. Samples can be completed in a few minutes and proper treatment can be recommended in a timely manner. Treatments for Clostridium spp. and coccidiosis can be done without delay and help minimize infection to other calves.

Organism	Age when signs observed	Fecal characteristics	Morbidity seen
E. coli *	1–5 days	Green or yellow	Very common
Clostridium *	2–21 days	Gray, with blood	Not often
Rotavirus * (viral)	4–15 days	Watery, no color	Common
Coronavirus * (viral)	7–30 days	Watery, no color	Common
Salmonella *	7–30 days	Powerful odor, with blood	Rare
Cryptospori- diosis	8–20 days	Watery, some straining. No response to treatment.	Common
Coccidiosis	Usually 21+ days	-	Common in runoff areas

Table 9: *Main diarrhea-causing organisms, age when signs are observed, and characteristics of feces.*[40] *Pre-calving vaccination of heifers or cows dramatically decreases the incidence of diseases marked with *.*

Remember, the times of infection correspond to the period when maternal antibodies are decreasing dramatically and the calf is trying to develop its immune system. *This is a critical period in calf survival* and attention must be directed to evaluating calf health during this time.

40. Sage Trail Veterinary Clinic handout, 2000.

Dehydration

A calf is approximately 70 percent water at birth, but loss of body fluids through diarrhea can produce rapid dehydration. Dehydration and the loss of certain electrolytes produce dramatic changes in the calf's body chemistry that can quickly lead to death.

The difference between moderate dehydration (5–6%) and severe dehydration (8–10%) is less than 1 liter of fluids in circulating blood. Severe diarrhea can cause 1 liter of fluid loss in only 1–2 hours, so immediate attention is essential.

The age of the calf when scours begins is an important consideration in its survival. With diarrhea in young calves, the younger the calf, the greater the percentage fluid loss, and therefore, the greater the chance of death.

Detecting dehydration

Dehydration can be evaluated by testing for skin or hide elasticity and examining clinical signs. A small difference in percentage of dehydration can be detected in this way. The recommended skin area to evaluate dehydration is from the middle of the neck, which is tented and twisted slightly, then let go to return to the original position.

Time to return to normal position	Evaluation	Other symptoms expected
2 seconds or less	Normal	-
5–6 seconds	Moderate dehydration (5–6%)	Depressed, weak, cold extremities, ataxic, eyes slightly sunken.
8 or more seconds	Severe dehydration (8–10%)	Calf if usually unable to stand.

Table 10: *Evaluating dehydration via skin examination of calves.*[41]

Treating moderate dehydration

At moderate dehydration of 5–6% calves are ataxic, weak, and cold in the extremities (ears, lips, and feet). The calf should be cared for to minimize heat loss. With fluid loss and dehydration, body heat loss is extreme, and normal body functions slow down, with shock and toxic effects resulting.

Dehydration can be overcome with simple fluids given by mouth *early* in the course of the disease. Dehydration will continue if aggressive action is not taken, and intravenous fluid treatment will become necessary.

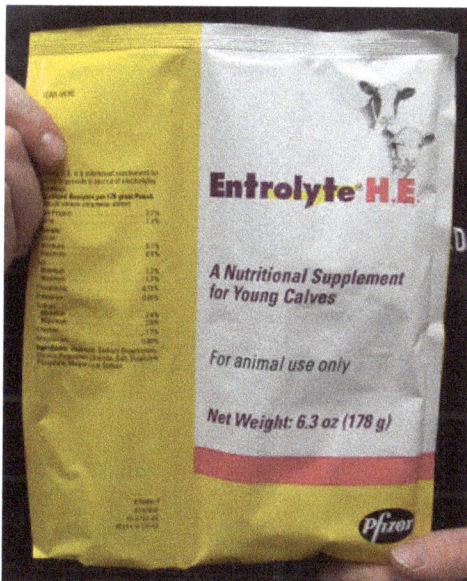

Image P03: *Oral electrolyte powder used for oral fluid replacement in calves.*

41. Data from Sage Trail Veterinary Clinic.

Treating severe dehydration

At 8–10% dehydration, fluid replacement is almost impossible to achieve by oral administration. IV treatment is necessary for success and restoring body function. Most calves at this state are unable to stand and are non-responsive. *This is a severe life-threatening crisis and immediate attention is necessary for success.*

Caution for preventing pneumonia is recommended at this point with body heat loss and risk of secondary infections. With inclement weather, diarrhea is followed by pneumonia, or diarrhea is a secondary problem with pneumonia calves.

E. coli and colibacilosis

E. coli

Escherichia coli (commonly called E. coli) occurs during the first 5–10 days of life. It usually causes green-yellow pasty diarrhea, and often indicates the presence of other stresses (this is critical especially in cold weather). Producers can eliminate the cause by doing pre-calving vaccination (approx. $1.25–1.50 per cow), and the disease has low mortality if treated properly using oral fluids and antibiotics for secondary pneumonia. Each case results in a loss of 10–14 lbs. at weaning (value $10–18), plus $3–5 of treatment costs.

E. coli is the most common cause of diarrhea in the first 5 days after birth, and is highly related to stress, poor colostrum intake, and unsanitary environmental conditions.

Though some people recommend obtaining a culture and sensitivity report, this advice is controversial, as contamination factors dilute the diagnostic capability and result in a false diagnosis in many cases.

Calves usually respond well if fluid intake is controlled by reversing fluid loss and correcting dehydration and acidosis. Up to 80–90% of producers vaccinate their cows 1–4 months prior to calving, with excellent results. Vaccination is inexpensive, average costs are $1–2 per cow vaccinated, depending on the product used. Considering the alternative, this management decision has a high economical return. E. coli scour products can be used with other combination scour products for greater range of control or prevention.

Colibacilosis

This refers to infection due to one or multiple serotypes of Escherichia coli, often causing septicemia and resulting in a poor prognosis. Many different serotypes of E. coli cause diarrheas and septicemias in calves under one week of age. *These conditions are directly due to inadequate amounts of colostrum, or untimely intake, or exposure of the pathogen before colostrum intake or absorption.*

Three types of E. coli are commonly associated with diarrheas, with the most common being the enterotoxigenic type. As the type states, these produce toxins (in fast-growth conditions) and are absorbed producing depression, inappetence, and secondary infections. Environmental challenges such as inclement weather add to the risk factors associated with colibacilosis.

Enterotoxic E. coli is the most common cause of acute mortality in week old calves.[42] These calves, usually because of energy loss and decreased nursing, have below-normal temperatures and require intensive treatment and care for several days, requiring labor and medical costs. Mortality is as high as 80%, and surviving calves often

---

42. www.VetsWeb.com

show arthritis and poor gain performance.[43] Infected calves need to be isolated from the other calves and treated aggressively.

The most common signs of colibacilosis are:

+ diarrhea in one-to-two-day-old calves,

+ depression,

+ lack of energy to suckle, and

+ dehydration and death within 48 hours.

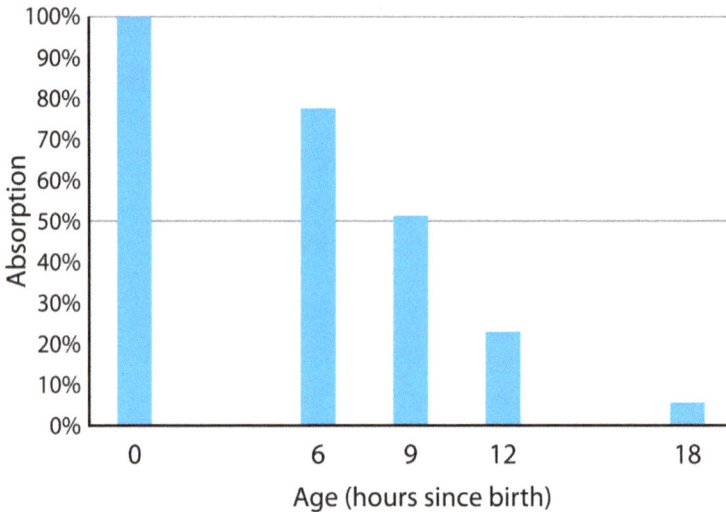

Figure 9 (repeated): Percent of immunoglobulin absorbed, by age in hours since birth. Colibacillosis calves are often the calves that have nursed or fed colostrum after 6 hours from birth, thus absorbing only a fraction of adequate levels of colostrum.

As the main defense against E. coli is passive transfer of immunity through colostrum, valuable calves should receive blood transfer

43. Sager, 2011.

from the dam (with immunoglobulins) for better chances of surviv-al. Rehydration therapy with intravenous antibiotic therapy is also necessary for success. Amoxicillin has been shown to be the most effective antimicrobial therapy in the past.[44]

In considering treatment, one must consider that the use of oral amoxicillin acts as an anti-microbial against normal intestinal floral as well as the infection. For this reason, IV treatment is recommend-ed rather than oral. A combination of injectable Nuflor and non-steroidal anti-inflammatory drug (NSAID) products have shown results for this author, but must be used aggressively and over 7–10 days treatment time.

There is a high correlation of septic colibacilosis calves that have failed to receive colostrum during the first few hours of life. They either ingest pathogens, or fail to receive adequate colostrum levels necessary for protection of pathogenic bacteria like the enterotoxic E. coli strains. *Blood taken from new-born calves during the first 2 weeks of life can indicate if adequate colostrum was absorbed if subjected to a refractometer analysis of total protein levels in serum.* This can be done at most veterinary clinics to evaluate if a calf had adequate colostrum intake after birth.

Clostridium complexes

This refers to clostridium perfringens type C and D. (Also known as C. perfringens or bloody scours.)

+ Most commonly seen at 4½-8 weeks of age, but can be seen at any age. Typically appears when the cow reaches maximum lactation, or when there is a change in feed that

44. Sager, 2011.

increases milk production suddenly. Colostridium per-fringes type C is more common than type D.

+ Can be controlled by nutritional management. Dropping protein by 20% can have quick success in reducing disease in calves. The disease is often seen when green grass starts; try changing from alfalfa to grass hays.

+ Look for blood-flecked, mucous-streaked, pasty diarrhea. A microscopic slide diagnosis by a veterinarian can identify the organism. This can be done easily in a veterinary office without sending the sample out for a laboratory diagnosis.

+ Is easily controlled and eliminated by vaccination at birth using a micro-encapsulated oil vaccine, such as Alpha 7 from Boehringer Ingleheim Pharmaceuticals.

+ Often causes sudden death in fast-growing calves. Usually the calves that are doing the best are affected by Colostridium perfringes type C.

+ Recommend prescription use of antitoxin, along with supportive treatment, to reduce gas in the intestinal tract.

+ Vaccination costs $0.75–1.00 per calf and is more effective than relying on passive colostrum protection without vaccination.

Common symptoms with this disease complex include diarrhea with gaseous bloating (bacterial cause) and abdominal pain, and discomfort (kicking at belly, tail lifting, distention) in the first 2–10 days. Often seen in calves nursing from cows that are fed higher0protein feeds, such as alfalfa hay. Toxin absorption in the small intestine can result in severe neurological signs and can kill the calf within hours.

Sudden death often occurs before diarrhea is noticed.

Recommendation: Do a necropsy when sudden death occurs. A necropsy is necessary for diagnosis of clostridium complexes after sudden death. Many times, the best value is the money spent on this necropsy. When in doubt, perform one.

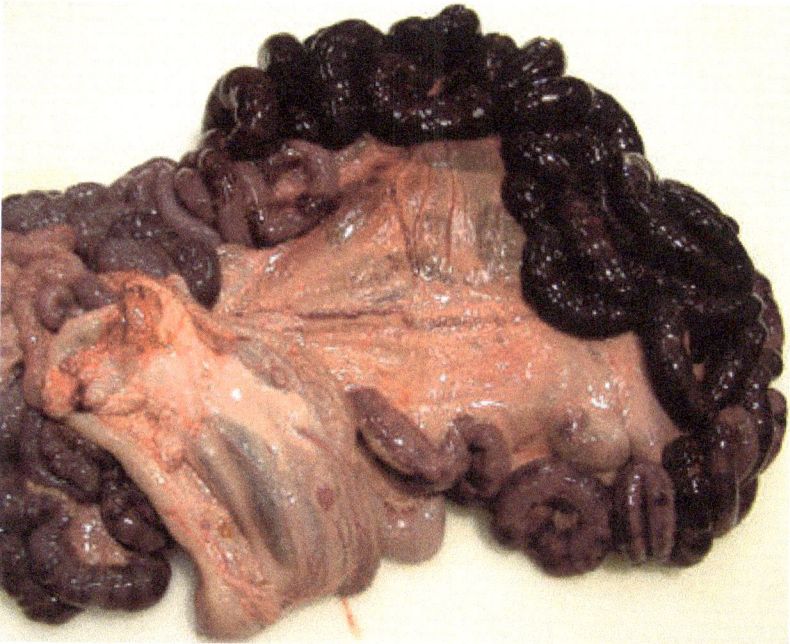

Image N01: Calf necropsy—small bowel examination. This calf died of Clostridium perfingens type C.[45]

When performing a necropsy, you will often see sloughed intestinal tissue in the diarrhea along with blood flecks. Toxins cause severe tissue necrosis, and as a result dead tissue is sloughed with the fecal material. This is very important as the new tissue cannot function as efficiently as the original intestinal tissue, in terms of absorption

45. Montana State Veterinary Diagnostic Laboratory slide, 2011.

of nutrients, as scarring takes place. This tissue change is permanent and can result in lost growth and performance later in life.

This disease can be diagnosed easily by a fecal smear stained to identify C. perfringens organisms. This disease is most commonly seen in herds with a high milking index and feeding lactating cows higher protein hays.

This disease is often seen in herds where genetic traits (traits selected for growth and milk production) increase susceptibility. This can be easily managed by controlling protein intake levels in lactating cows, by pre-calving vaccination of cows, or by post-calving vaccination of calves. The most common approach is to use an oil-based vaccine in the calf at birth.

Over the past twenty years, because of the introduction of clostridia vaccines given at birth or during the first week of life, there has been a dramatic reduction in the incidence of this devastating disease complex. These vaccines are micro-encapsulated oil-based products designed for slow absorption and long-term antibody duration. They are widely used and are very successful. Most products are priced in the $0.75–0.80 range per dose.

For acute disease treatment, Clostridium C and D antitoxin is used to reverse the toxin production of the fast-growing bacteria, to avoid those toxins being absorbed in the small intestine. This product is given subcutaneously (after warming up the product so it can be absorbed faster) per directions in multiple areas.

Colstridium Type A

Recently, a type A Clostridium infection causing similar clinical signs has been identified. In some areas a separate Clostridium Type

A vaccine needs to be used at birth (in most cases, this is better than giving it to the cow). This helps to prevent sudden death in calves under 3–4 weeks of age. (Future vaccine products will have all three types, C, D, and A, included in the same product.)

The difference in identifying Type A from the more common C and D types is that a larger area of intestine is infected, causing more blood loss and more toxin absorption. Ranchers should contact their veterinarian concerning this new Clostridium disease.

Viral diarrhea complexes

Rotavirus and Coronavirus infections are the most common viral causes of diarrhea.

- A common sign is watery diarrhea, *often not seen on the tail or ground because of the extremely watery consistency of feces.* Be careful not to miss this sign.

- Typically appears at 5–14 days of age, most commonly in calves born to heifers or second-calf cows.

- Can be controlled through pre-calving vaccination. Cost is typically $3.50–4.00 per cow, 1–3 months before calving.

- Calves dehydrate very rapidly because of greatly increased fluid loss. They need immediate fluid therapy, consisting of IV and supportive care by a veterinary professional.

- These diseases are very costly, as intestinal tissue does not repair well, and malabsorption problems during the growth phase results in calves that are 30–100 lbs. lighter at weaning, typically translating to a loss of $50–200 per incident.

Rotavirus is almost always seen from 5–14 days of age, and especially in calves born to young heifers or cows, as the virus is shed from the dam and infects the calf. Rotavirus is the most common diarrhea of the viral scour groups.

The most striking physical signs are the watery diarrhea and the rapid dehydration. Because the diarrhea is watery, it is often missed as it does not stick to the tail where it could be observed later. This disease calls for immediate treatment with oral fluids and replacement energy.

Commercial vaccines are available for the dam; these are given 1–3 months before calving. It is recommended to vaccinate the first-calf and second-calf heifers during normal conditions, and to vaccinate the entire cow herd when viral scours is diagnosed in the entire herd (not just in the calves from heifers).

This disease requires immediate attention, as dehydration is severe and quick to cause problems. Remember *calves die of dehydration, not just from the infection of the virus.* This is more critical than with bacterial scours. The calf will respond with treatment and replacement fluids, and can recover from the virus without secondary problems occurring.

Coronavirus signs are almost identical to Rotavirus, and are usually seen at a later age, although there is some overlap in the ages when the two diseases are usually diagnosed. Treatment, costs, and prevention are the same as for Rotavirus.

This disease represents the second most common viral diarrhea problem in young beef calves. It is seen less often than Rotavirus, yet shows the same clinical signs and is just as severe in causing dehydration. This disease usually is seen later than rotavirus, between

10–30 days of age. Remember, it is not the virus that kills, *it is the dehydration that kills.*

Again, vaccination can easily help prevent any viral scour problems.

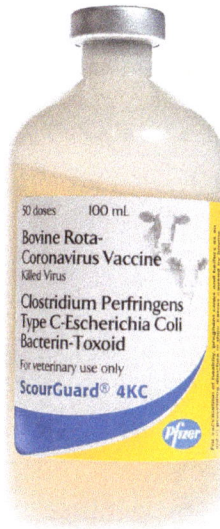

Image P04: *ScourGuard 4KC by Pfizer Animal Health. (Bovine Rota-Coronavirus Vaccine.)*

In acute outbreaks, an oral vaccine (Calf Guard) given to the calf at birth can be used to block the receptor sites of the virus from attaching to the intestinal villi. Mixed results have been noted. It is the author's impression that the sooner the calf is treated with the oral vaccine before colostrum nursing, the better the response to the product. After nursing, the vaccine does not seem to protect as well.

Salmonella

Salmonella dublin, Salmonella typhimurium, and other Salmonella serotypes (>286 serotypes) are less-common (but important) diarrhea-causing diseases that have the following characteristics:

+ Extremely depressed calves, with bloody, mucous diarrhea carrying a strongly offensive odour

+ Most severe in terms of depression and greatest risk as a zoonotic (animal-to-human transfer).

+ Often seen with poor-energy nutrition, and extremely muddy or unsanitary conditions

+ Almost no good treatment, as Salmonella serotypes are resistant to most antibiotics. Success requires excellent supportive treatment over a long period of time.

+ Vaccination pre-calving in problem herds can be effective and costs $1.50–2.00 per cow. However, there are only a couple of good vaccines commercially available.

+ Significant financial impact because the disease has high mortality and is highly infective. Cows that have not calved should be moved to a new area.

This disease complex is often seen with energy deficiency problems in baby calves, and is severe, resulting in very sick calves. Calves can be infected within hours of birth from contaminated udders or surroundings. The disease is most common between 4–24 days of age. Depression and weakness are more severe than in other diarrheas. Salmonella often follows after calves have been exposed to very unsanitary conditions, and often is transferred by rodent-infested feeds or environmental contamination. Clinical signs often show up as mucous-stained bloody scours, with diarrhea that is green to dark green in color, and characteristically has a strongly offensive odor that distinguishes this disease from other diarrheas.

This disease often results in very sick calves with small amounts of diarrhea, sometimes thick with tissues from the colon or rectal area that have been sloughed with diarrhea.

Warning: Salmonella can transfer to humans, with severe consequences.

Salmonella is a human zoonotic. Producers must take serious care not to contaminate themselves while treating this disease. Sick calves are known to shed as many as one billion Salmonella organisms per day.[46] *The use of a sick pen is not recommended.*

Control of this serious disease is much like other recommended disease control programs:

1. Eliminate the source of infection.

2. Remove the calf from the contaminated environment.

3. Increase the non-specific and specific immunity of the calf.

4. Improve the environment by reducing stress.

5. Specific treatment for the calf.

---

46. Smith, 2009.

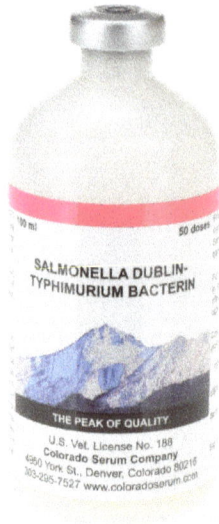

Image P05: *Salmonella vaccine (Colorado Serum Company).*

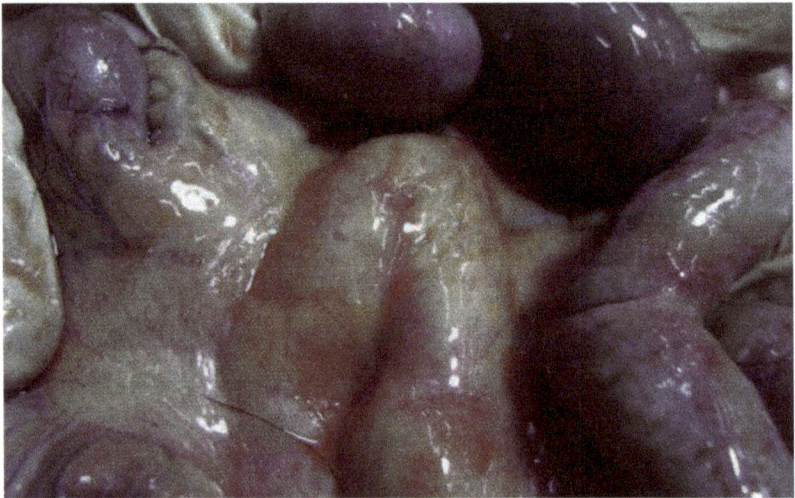

Image N02: *Necropsy of a calf that died from Salmonella, showing typical signs.*[47]

47. *Veterinary Clinics* Volume 25: Number 1, March 2009.

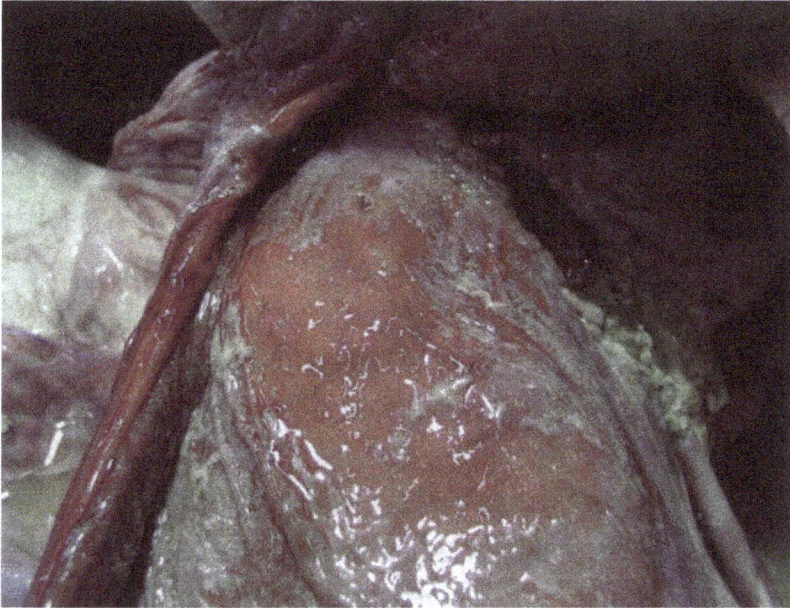

Image N03: *Additional salmonella necropsy photo.*[48]

Cryptosporidiosis

Cryptosporidiosis parvum and other Cryptosporidiosis serotypes have the following characteristics:

+ Opportunists that appear with other diarrheas.

+ Zoonotic infection transfer to humans.

+ Usually appears at 2–4 weeks of age.

+ Causes malabsorption of nutrients due to diarrhea.

+ Oocysts appearing in fecal sample can be used for diagnosis.

48. *Veterinary Clinics* Volume 25: Number 1, March 2009.

- No specific prescription fluids or supportive treatments.

- Coccidiostactic products can be of help.

Protozoan in origin, Cryptosporidiosis is an opportunist, which means it usually follows a previous scour problem rather than being the primary problem. It does not have any specific treatment. This organism infects the lining of the small intestine and is zoonotic: it will transfer to humans of all ages. It is most commonly a problem in newborn calves. It is immunosuppressive and infects the intestinal cells by spreading internally (intracellular). It can develop in as little as 12–14 hours, producing large numbers of organisms in several days.

Diarrhea and abdominal cramping are clinical signs, producing fluid loss, dehydration, and electrolyte imbalances. Billions of organisms can be shed from a single calf in a few days, which makes this disease highly infective. Ionophores such as Rumensin (Lasalocid) and Moneinsin can be used, but the treatment dosages are very close to toxic levels. The most common recommendation is to flush large amounts of fluids orally. Production of a vaccine has been considered for years, but protozoan organisms are most difficult to incorporate into antigen production for vaccines, and therefore future production is doubtful.

These are Protozoan parasites, containing up to 14 species, and are common in all mammals, birds, and fish. Cryptosporidiosis is an uncommon disease in cattle, but when diagnosed is severe and serious in producing economic problems. Common signs are persistent diarrhea that is non-responsive to any treatment, a watery diarrhea accompanied by some straining.

This disease can often be devastating. Because of the calf's young age, lack of resistance, and typical presence of other stresses, Cryptosporidiosis can be a killer through dehydration and secondary bacterial enteritis. The organism is common to the intestinal tracts of cows and studies show organism shedding during pre-calving is increased toward calves and clinical signs appear as early as five days of age.[49] Because of the protozoal characteristics, infection is by fecal contamination of millions of oocysts in water or feed. Oocysts are resistant to disinfectants and antibiotics (in fact, this type of treatment may increase severity, because it decreases the number of competing organisms). Success is generally the result of intensive oral treatment of electrolytes and fluids, and essentially flushing the organism out of the intestinal tract.

It must be considered that infection may recur from one year to another. as the organism will persist over long periods of time. Freezing and drying will kill the organism, but remember, *the cow is often the carrier*, especially in first-calving and second-calving cows. Calves with lower colostrum intake are more susceptible to infection and pass larger numbers of oocysts after infection.

Age resistance is not a factor in calves the way it is in other mammals, and often problems occur when ranchers are about ready to turn out for grass. This disease problem seems to be more common than it was twenty years ago. Even with successful treatment, long-term intestinal absorption is decreased, and weaning weights are affected as a result. There are no characteristics on necropsy that point to Cryptosporidia infection, but large numbers of the organism can be seen on slide swabs of large intestine tissue. Remember, in cold weather the rancher must give energy along with electrolytes, or the calf will be in a negative energy balance and "crash".

49. Radostits, 2007.

Typical cotton ear swabs kept moist in a container can be transported to a veterinary clinic, swabbed on glass slides, and stained to see most organisms easily. This is a simple diagnosis that can be made without the cost and time needed for shipment to a laboratory. This will give you an initial idea that will help minimize shedding to other calves if the test is positive.

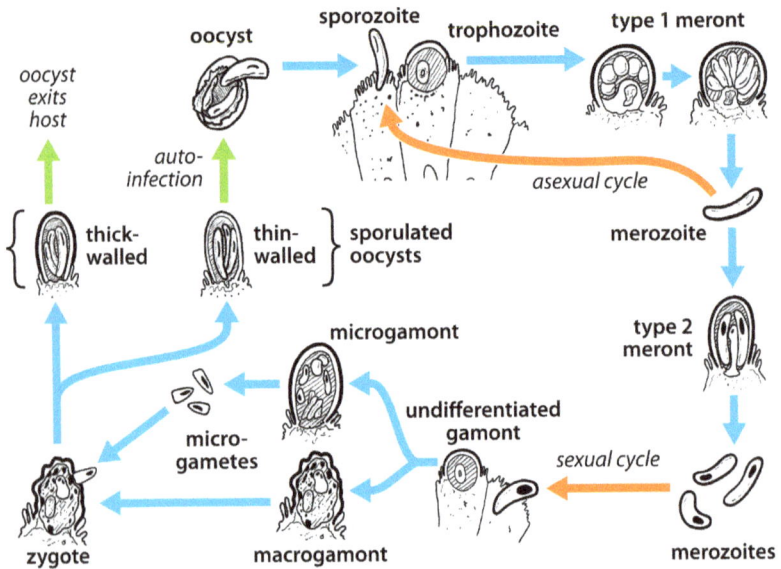

Figure 13: The complex life cycle of Cryptosporidiosis.[50]

Coccidiosis

Characteristics of Coccidiosis (Emeria spp. and Isospora spp. being the most common):

+ High rate of occurrence, but with low mortality except when complicated by secondary infections.

50. http://www.dpd.cdc.gov/dpdx/html/frames/a-f/cryptosporidiosis/
body_cryptosporidiosis_life_cycle_lrg.htm

+ Most common in two-to-four-week-old calves in crowded conditions.

+ Transmitted by infected udders or pooling of contaminated water.

+ Straining with diarrhea. Blood can be seen on top of diarrhea because of straining to defecate.

+ Microscopic identification of oocysts in fecal sample.

+ Treat with fluids and Corid (coccidiostat) drench orally.

+ Remove infected calves or move non-infected herd from the contaminated source.

A disease caused by a protozoan parasite that produces intra-cellular infection in the cells lining the terminal end of the colon. Infection rates are high in crowded conditions, with severe diarrhea in younger calves. Transmitted by fecal contamination of all livestock species, and commonly seen around moist areas like water tanks and puddles of runoff, which are common sites of contamination for infection.

Cold weather is a common precursor to infection, and other stresses can be too. The normal animal has small numbers of coccidia present, and sheds oocysts regularly, allowing infection to persist.

The most common finding is many calves in a small or crowded area showing diarrhea. The diarrhea is usually blood-tinged or shows streaks of red blood. The blood is not digested or dark, because the infection occurs in the last part of the colon or large bowel. Usually straining is seen with the diarrhea.

Normally not seen in normal pasture conditions, except when water supplies are contaminated or calves drink from puddles from water tank overflows, or from contaminated puddles which have large numbers of oocysts. Clinical infection disappears with drying weather and conditions.

Control is achieved by using oral coccidiostats and controlling population density to minimize infection rates. Immunity will develop in time, and the disease rarely infects older animals, except at weaning under stress conditions or infection opportunities.

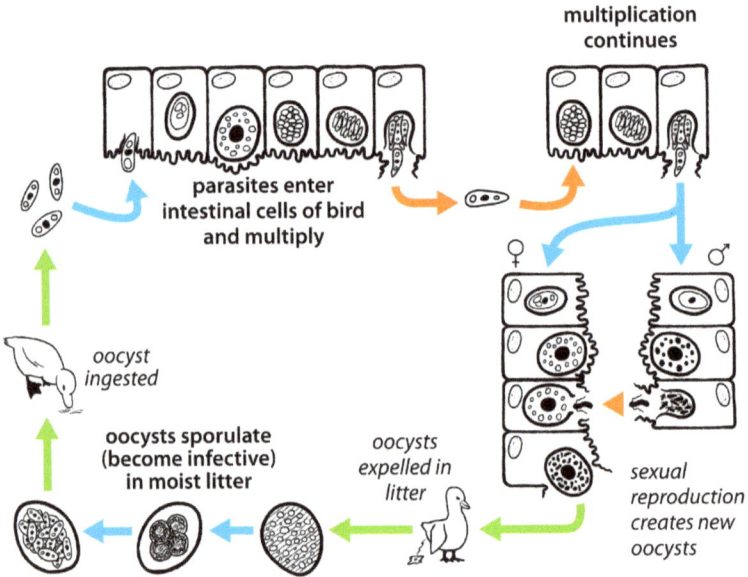

Figure 14: The life cycle of Coccidiosis.[51]

---

51. Adapted from Saxonet.

Preventing diarrhea: colostrum, vaccination, and other tips

Past research has indicated that many scour cases can be directly related to lack of colostrum intake by the newborn calf. A calf that is well-mothered and consumes 1-to-2 quarts of colostrum in the first few hours after birth absorbs a higher level of antibodies and is far less susceptible to scours and other calf diseases. The difference can be as dramatic as one tenth the incidence, compared to calves that receive inadequate quality or quantity of colostrum.

The most common cause of diarrhea is bacterial, which can be caused by contamination from the udder of the cow. A clean area at calving time is important to prevent bacterial scours transmitted via udder contamination.

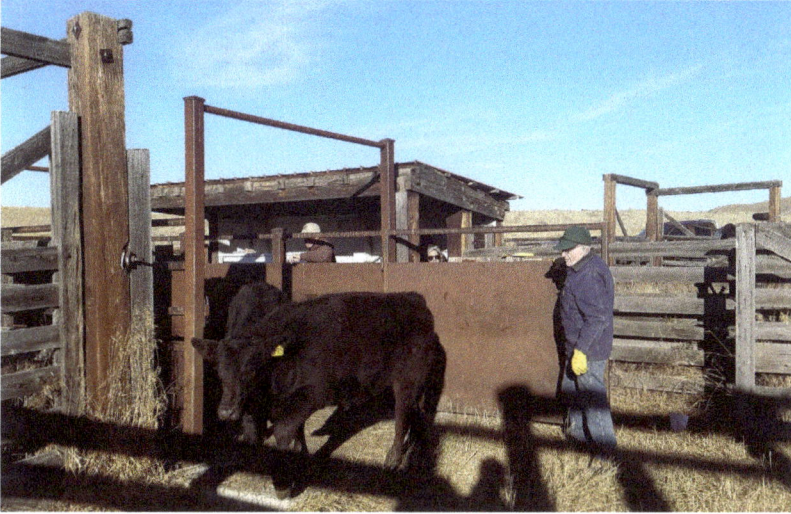

4

Pneumonia and BRD

Respiratory disease is a constant challenge for beef producers. It causes nearly 25% of all pre-weaning deaths. Treatment therapy and preventative vaccine programs have improved calf health, yet the seriousness of the problem remains vast.

Losses from respiratory complications are estimated to be *over $2.2 billion yearly* in the United States.[52]

52. Radostits, 2007.

Unlike in calf diarrhea, where treatment or fluid replacement can buy time for the normal healing response to take place, the loss of respiratory function cannot be overcome, and death results in a relatively short time.

Defenses of the bovine respiratory system

The respiratory system of a cow is defended by a complex system of physiological, chemical, and immunological agents that are involved in a highly complex, yet efficient, interaction that actively minimizes infections every minute of every day.

These defenses include the following:

- **Mucous secretion**, which traps invading organisms and is increased by neurological stimulation caused by foreign proteins coming into contact with cells responsible for secretion, which are found under the mucous membranes. (The coloration of mucous is the result of chemicals from leukocytes that oxidize invading organisms, as well as dust and environmental factors.)

- **Sneezing**, a response initiated by mast cells under the mucus membranes of respiratory tissues when those membranes are inflamed

- **Coughing**, which eliminates excess mucous, infectious organisms, and inflammatory exudates

- **Mucociliary transport**, which creates upward movement of any inhaled bacteria and viruses across mucus-covered areas, resulting in the common snot formed at the nares of calves (these secretions are a good sign, not a bad one)

- **The anatomy of the respiratory system**, which filters

and traps organisms before they can enter the deeper respiratory tissues

+ **Local secretion of Immunoglobulin A antibodies** from mucous membranes

+ **The adaptive immune system**, which attacks any organisms that pass by the innate immune system

Pneumonia and BRD result when these defenses are unable to prevent infection.

Pneumonia

Pneumonia refers to inflammation of the pulmonary system. Clinical signs include rapid and shallow breathing, changes in depth and character of respiratory movements, coughing, abnormal sounds accompanying breathing, wetness around the mouth from rapid air movement, depression, and toxemia.

This inflammatory damage causes permanent tissue loss, decreased alveolar gas exchange, a chronic disease state, and resulting decreased longevity.

In the upper Great Plains of the United States, calf pneumonia accounts for more than 50% of all sickness.

What causes pneumonia?

Pneumonia can be caused by a variety of viruses and bacteria. When these organisms are inhaled and defeat the normal defense mechanisms of the cow's respiratory system, the resulting infection causes pneumonia. Bacterial pneumonia produces wet cough reflexes, which are different from the drier cough observed with viral infections.

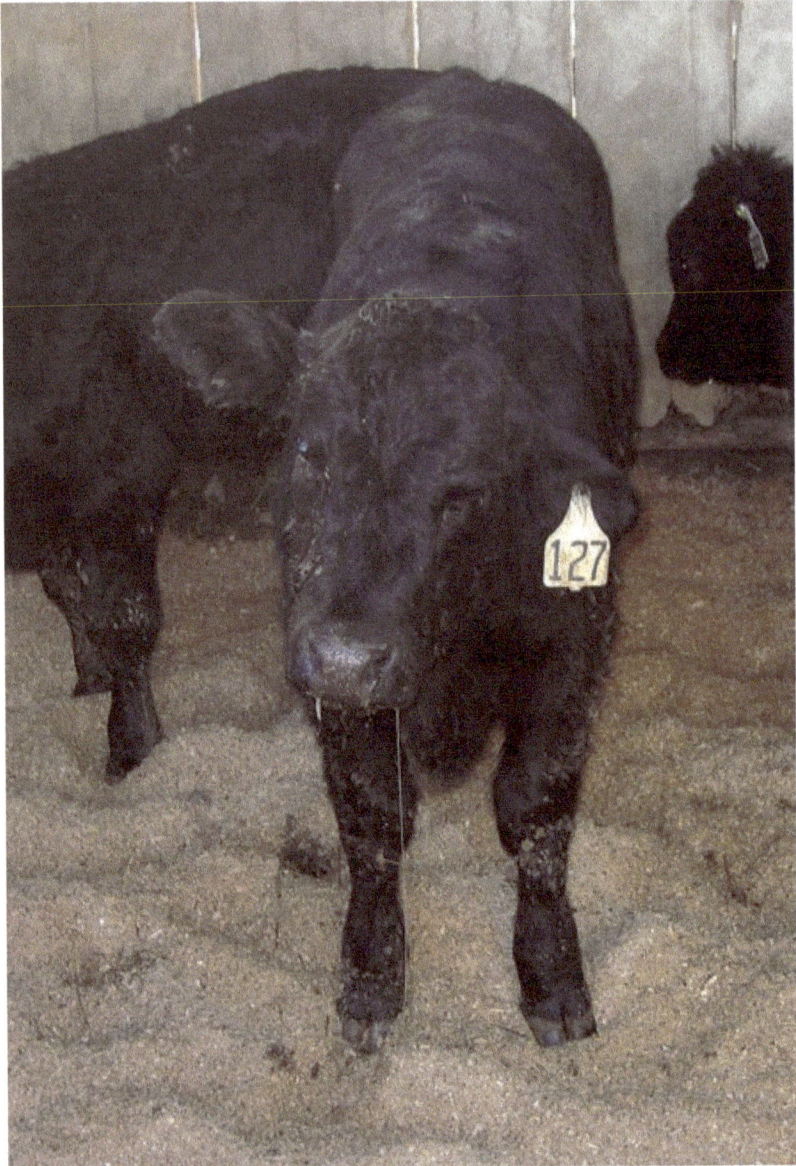

Image D01: *Calf with pneumonia. Note drooling, dropped ears, and lethargy.*[53]

---

53.   Picture courtesy of Virginia Extension Service.

Susceptibility to pneumonia is determined by many factors, including genetics and the calf's resistance to infection by the agents that cause pneumonia.[54]

Experience will allow the rancher to observe that pneumonia problems follow stress from diarrhea, chilled conditions, or poor colostrum absorption. Disease severity is directly influenced by the infectious organism involved, environmental conditions, and the immune system response of the calf.

Why is pneumonia so common?

The answer is complex, but no other factor is as important as the anatomy of the bovine lung.

In cows, the area of lung volume per body weight is smaller than in other mammals. Their anatomy is also more compartmentalized than other livestock. As a result, cattle have a smaller gaseous exchange capacity, are often close to hypoxia, and have more contaminated air flow patterns. Their airways can become occluded by less of an immune response than other mammals. These differences predispose them to pulmonary problems.[55]

Environmental conditions, physiological demands, and microbial stresses all affect respiratory stress much more in bovines than in other mammals, and because of this, infection and disease is more likely. Conditions such as increased temperature, humidity, or stress can lead to major complications.

---

54. Smith, 2005.

55. Radostits, 2007.

The effect of weather

The stress of weather during normal calving periods is also a factor in causing pneumonia. Weather-related stresses require larger energy resources, which often cannot be supplied by the cow's milk, resulting in disease problems.

Bovine Respiratory Disease (BRD)

Bovine respiratory disease (BRD) is the most common and costly disease affecting beef cattle in the world. It is a bacterial infection that causes pneumonia and can be fatal.

BRD accounts for approximately 75% of feedlot disease and 50–70% of all feedlot deaths.[56] The majority of deaths due to BRD occur shortly after arrival to the feedlot or within the first 45 days.[57] In fact, about 91% of calves diagnosed with BRD are diagnosed within the first 27 days after arrival.[58]

Bovine Respiratory Disease causes an estimated $800 million to $900 million in economic losses from death, reduced feed efficiency, and treatment costs annually.[59]

Veterinary medical costs attributable to the treatment of BRD are substantial, and the economic impacts of BRD on carcass merit and meat quality further increase the economic costs. Medicine costs accounted for 21% of the decrease, while 79% was attributable to lower carcass weight (8.4% lower) and lower quality grade (24.7% more USDA Standard quality grade carcasses).

56. Edwards, 1996; Galyean et al., 1999; Loneragan et al., 2001

57. Edwards, 1996; Loneragan et al., 2001

58. BUHMAN ET AL., 2000

59. CHIRASE AND GREENE, 2001

BRD alone is estimated to cost feedlot management over $500 million annually even with preconditioning of calves and new health programs in place.[60] A Texas A&M Ranch-to-Rail Study found BRD morbidity accounted for 8% higher production costs, not including losses related to decreased performance.[61] They found cattle with BRD had a 3% decrease in gain compared with healthy cattle and cost the program $111.38 per sick animal. Snowder et al (2006) estimated economic losses in a 1,000-head feedlot from BRD infection to be approximately $13.90 per animal due to lower gains and treatment costs.

The total health costs in beef cattle production in the United States from sickness and loss of production are projected to be greater than $2.2 billion annually.[62] An estimated 25% of all calf deaths before weaning can be attributed to BRD.[63] BRD is the largest single cause of mortality reported in feedlots and accounts for more than 28% of all beef calf mortality problems.[64]

What causes BRD?

Calves are constantly breathing microbes into their lower respiratory tract. Normally, these microbes are either removed by the normal mucociliary transport mechanism as nasal secretions, defeated by the cow's immune defenses, or because of the anatomy of the lung never penetrate to the tissues below the large airways.

However, if the calf is already suffering from other problems, there

---

60. TAYLOR ET AL, 2010

61. GRIFFIN ET AL., 1995

62. Jacaub, 1984; Confer, 2005; Radostits, 2007.

63. USDA NAHMS, 2007.

64. Van Eenennaam, 2011.

are various ways these microbes can invade the respiratory system and be "triggered" to undergo rapid growth, leading to BRD.

A pre-existing viral or bacterial infection is the most common trigger. (In particular, Mannheimia haemolytica.)[65] This existing stress on the cow's immune system allows the BRD microbes to take hold.

Existing local tissue damage is commonly seen in the form of viral organisms that procure bacterial pneumonia. The virus damages the respiratory tissue lining, allowing the entry of bacterial organisms that would normally be filtered away or removed.

Interrupted circulation and fluid-filled alveoli can both occur due to inflammation that is already present from other causes.

Stresses and energy deficit also contribute to development of BRD.

Once the microbes penetrate past the large airways and take hold, BRD follows.

Additional effects of BRD

Because of the anatomy of bovine lung tissue, and the complex immune system response to infection, much of the affected lung tissue is destroyed permanently. This results in long term loss of production, a chronic disease state, and reduced longevity.

Detecting BRD

Many times, the most difficult part of maintaining calf health is to identify whether a calf is sick. Almost always these problems are multi-factorial diseases, as a mammal's inflammatory stimulus to infection initially is at the cellular level. Important chemokines are

---

65. Smith, 2001; 2005.

released from regulatory immune cells within the tissues of the body. Some of the most important and fastest to react are the immune "surveillance cells" underneath the skin, inside the mucosal linings of the respiratory tract, or beneath mucosa tissues of the intestinal tissues. A complicated immune system response that identifies foreign proteins and molecules that trigger a fascinating, complicated immune reflex takes place immediately and initiates the protection processes of the immune system. Within minutes, important chemokines and cytokines are released to travel to the hypothalamus in the brain; this stimulates the hypothalamus to increase the body temperature, which facilitates immune system chemicals to act more efficiently and to hinder growth of microbial invaders.

One of the first and most useful steps that need to be taken is to evaluate body temperature, as this will be the first initial sign of any inflammatory response. A simple thermometer is adequate and can be easily carried in coveralls or a saddle bag. It is critical not to stress the calf when trying to evaluate temperature, as even a little stress can increase normal body temperature, leading to false readings and a false diagnosis. A mild stress will raise body temperature by 1–2 degrees and, most importantly, cause additional stress to the calf and delay the immune response.

A calf's normal temperature should be 101.5–102.2 with no additional stress. This can be an invaluable sign for beginning infection or any inflammatory condition. As simple as this may sound, it is one of the best methods to answer the question "is my calf sick?". Have any treatment already dosed and ready to administer so to minimize additional handling of the calf that would result in added stress. This is the critical time to answer the question: "is my calf sick, can I treat it successfully, or do I need to consult my veterinarian?"

One of the most important lessons is the fact that "almost anything done early is much better than a lot of things done later". Documented cases show repeatedly that early detection and treatment not only saves time and energy, but also affects the pocketbook.

Cowboy tip: A calf that is sick for one day can cost you more than $25 (not counting treatment costs) at weaning or shipping, due to reduced growth and weight gains during the summer period, as infected tissue requires both energy and time to heal, resulting in poor growth and performance.

Treating Pneumonia and BRD

The use of antimicrobials has been an important and effective treatment that can produce desired results when started early in the disease course. The longer that the disease has been present and the more involved it is, the greater the difficulty and lower the efficacy of treatment. Because of the anatomy, the inflammatory reactions, and the environmental factors, pneumonia can be difficult to treat, and often is a large factor influencing future growth and production. Calf pneumonia will affect gain and carcass traits in the feedlot and performance will decrease and carcass value will decrease at slaughter a year later.

It is the author's experience that newer antibiotics, although more expensive, have given faster response and better results in avoiding weight losses, and are therefore of better value in the long run. For a few dollars more, better results can produce more than a $25.00 return in weaning weights. Newer antibiotics are designed for faster absorption, higher blood and tissue levels specific for inflammatory tissues, and can save labor by acting for several days. This reduces stress on the calf and provides for an increased success rate.

Product	Administration	Cost / 100lbs. per dose
Nuflor (*florfenicol*)	Intra-muscular 3mL / 100 lbs. / 48 hrs	$1.00
Draxxin (*tulathromycin*)	Subcutaneous 1.5 mL / 100 lbs. (lasts for 10 days)	$1.10
Micotil (*tilmicosin*)	Subcutaneous 2 mL / 100 lbs. (lasts for 4 days)	$2.25
Zactran (*gamithromycin*)	Subcutaneous 2 mL / 100 lbs. (lasts for 10 days)	$1.80
Zuprevo (*tildipirosin*)	Subcutaneous 1 mL / 100 lbs.	$1.00

Table 11: *Economics of antimicrobial products used for treatment of pneumonia.*

Be careful using older-generation antibiotics, such as tetracyclines, as the common BRD microbe has mutated and acquired a resistance. Many times, these products do not work well, and time is lost trying them before the producer realizes the animal is not responding. By this time, the disease process has advanced and caused chronic lung tissue damage that cannot be repaired, will affect growth and performance, and creates the risk of a chronic condition that will not respond to any treatment process.

The choice of an antibiotic is often based on the veterinarian's previous knowledge and experience on the farm, and experience from results of similar cases recently. Licensed products for the treatment of respiratory disease in bovines include: Florfenicol, fluoroquinolones, oxytetracycline, Tilmicosin (Mycotil), Draxxin (tulathromyicin), Zactran, and Zuprevo, which is also one of the macrolides form of antibiotics.

In addition to antimicrobials, ancillary therapy should be used to provide analgesia, stimulate nursing and reduce inflammation and pyrexia. Newer non-corticosteroid products (Banamine or Flunixamine) provide anti-inflammatory effects by blocking cytokine production as a result of inflammation. Corticosteroids and non-steroidal anti-inflammatory drugs (NSAIDs) represent the most commonly used ancillary therapies. The potential disadvantage of corticosteroids is their unselective suppression of inflammation, to the extent that the immune response, in particular macrophage infiltration that is vital to controlling infection, is also suppressed. NSAIDs act on the inflammatory reactive chemical cascade in a more selective manner, thus avoiding the potential immune suppression that is unwanted and harmful to the newborn calf.

NSAIDs are also analgesic and antipyretic, meaning they lower fever and help increase appetite necessary for fluid intake. Other ancillary treatments have been used for the treatment of pneumonia; these include antihistamines and expectorants; their use in practice is limited mostly by cost, availability, and the need for a veterinary license for purchase and use.

A personal viewpoint is that the use of these products decreases inflammation, including fever, and will promote the calf to nurse quicker than not using the products, often keeping the calf better-hydrated and preventing the need for drenching with electrolytes.

Basic animal husbandry using proper straw bedding is ideal for post-treatment, as energy reserves are decreased, feed intake is minimal, and dehydration is a concern. Straw, or any way for the animal to "warm up" or conserve heat in colder weather, is recommended, and is more important than many producers might suspect.

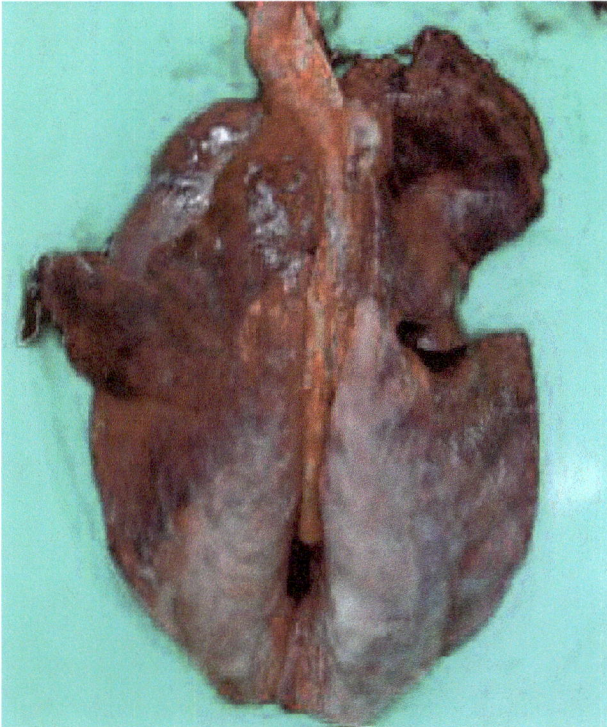

Image N04: *Bovine lung necropsy. This calf died from pneumonia. The necropsy shows acute congestion and a lack of normal tissue for air exchange. This diseased lung shows the consolidation and inflammation (reddened areas) of central tissues that are common signs of calf pneumonia. Normal lung tissue is visible as the white tissue toward the bottom of the image.*[66]

66. Potter, T. *UK Vet* Volume 12 Number 1, January 2007

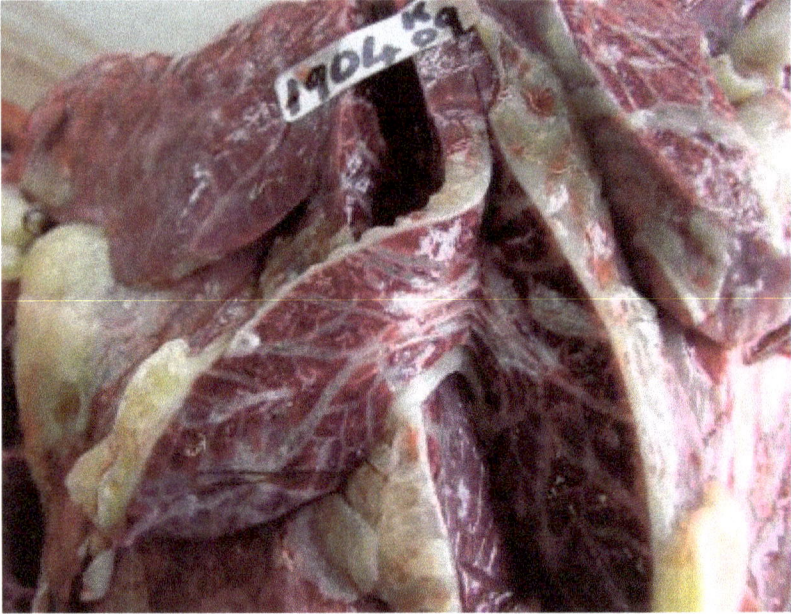

Image N05: *Necropsy of lung tissue. This calf died of Mannheimia hemolytica infection (BRD). Note the large amount of fibrin on the surface of the lung, which is typical of an M. hemolytica infection.*[67]

Why are Pneumonia and BRD such persistent problems?

Scientific data cannot explain why morbidity and mortality are similar to 50 years ago, even with advances in pharmaceutical technologies and advances in animal health.[68] In recent decades, we as veterinarians have seen more calf pneumonias than we did thirty years ago. The same problems are seen in feedlot production, even with a

67. http://www.agriculture.gov.ie/animalhealthwelfare/laboratoryservices/regionalveterinarylaboratoryreports/rvlmonthlyreports2009/april2009rvlmonthlyreport/

68. White, 2011.

better understanding of the disease process, better preventative recommendations, and better treatment products now than in the past. There is a distinct trend, evident since 1994, of increasing mortality from respiratory disease among cattle in feedlots, although the reasons have not been identified.[69]

Research is constantly being performed to confront the challenge of BRD. Newer antibiotics will continue to be developed as this area of bovine pharmacology is huge, being driven by the economics of the industry. The incidence of stress that predisposes post-weaning cows to BRD, caused by weaning, transportation, and interrupted feed intake, is high, leading to this economic pressure.

69. Radostits, 2007.

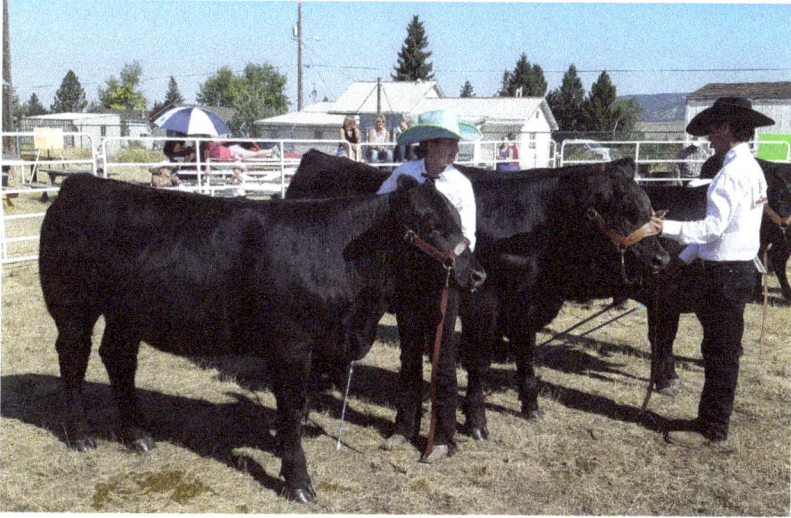

5

Preventive Health Recommendations

Key goals in management for prevention

The three goals of your management practices for preventive health should be biosecurity, increasing resistance, and treating individual animals.

Biosecurity refers to your efforts to prevent disease-causing organisms from entering your ranch. Do not buy infection.

Increasing resistance is accomplished not only through vaccination, but also through increasing the ability of the animal to respond to potential infections, mainly by increased nutrition.

Treating individual animals includes detecting and responding to specific problems, as well as removing the infected animal from susceptible herd mates.

Basic Immunology

The immune system starts to develop early in fetal development, beginning with the fetal liver (before birth), then the thymus and bone marrow after birth. In cattle, immune system growth is seen for the first eight months after birth, before the calf is finally "mature" in its ability to respond. Cells responsible for phagocytosis of foreign material are not in high numbers for a serious challenge until eight months.

Remember that the placental tissue of cattle does not permit transfer of antibodies to the fetus, therefore requiring that immune transfer be entirely from the intake of colostrum proteins in a timely manner. The bovine immune system is a product of adaptation through millions of years, is highly complex, and demands the ability of the calf to nurse within hours of birth for immune system success. For protection of the newborn calf, both passive immunity (colostrum immunoglobulins) and active immune system response are needed to respond to infection challenges.

Terms used in immunology

Vaccine antigenic mass or strength is the amount or quantity of antigen or "infection units" that is recognized by the immune system. It depends on the type of antigen, since the immune system responds very differently to each type. Some viral vaccines require millions or organisms per ml, while some vaccines that contain toxins require a much smaller amount or numbers for immune system stimulation to occur.

Local immunity is the development and containment of specific antibodies at the tissue surface (mucosa) or immediately beneath the mucosal surface. This is the first line of defense in the immune system.

Almost 70% of the total bovine immune system is near the intestinal mucosa, in structures called Peyer's patches that contain massive lymphoid tissue. The jejunum and ileum contain Peyer's patches that are considered the "immune sensors" of the intestine, and are important for immune protection at mucosal surfaces, as well as for the induction of mucosal immune responses in the intestine.

Humoral immunity is measured by the specific amount or number of antibodies that appear in circulating blood.

Recognition of an antigen (or foreign protein or substance) is the interaction and recognition of the foreign antigen or substance by specific immune cells found in circulating blood, as in white blood cells. This stimulates a cascade of specific cells through a very complex cellular interaction requiring 10 days to 2 weeks of time from the first exposure.

Memory is described as the ability for the immune system (both humoral and cell-mediated) to recognize previous exposure and respond quickly and specifically to another "exposure". *This is the goal of vaccination.*

Cell-mediated immunity occurs normally at the local tissue level and is the first line of defense in infections that cause inflammation (heat, color, swelling, and pain). It refers to specific phagocytic cells that engulf foreign proteins and compounds, so they can either be killed or transported to the lymph node for processing to become a template or key for specific antibody production. This response cannot be measured, unlike antibody levels, which can be measured through titers.

Vaccination response is determined by many factors, such as antigen specificity, administration route (subcutaneous vs. intramuscular), combination of antigen products, and added stress at vaccination.

Most commonly, antigen proteins stimulate good response as viruses are usually very specific and easy for the immune system to respond to, compared to bacteria that have many complex proteins or sub-particles that are needed for antigen presentation to cells for antibody secretion. In simple terms, the simpler and larger the antigen substrate or protein, the easier the immune system responds to stimulation.

Vaccine route of administration, such as nasal vs. injectable. Nasal administration causes a cellular local response, which mimics a more natural infection pattern and produces a much different response than a subcutaneous route, where the vaccine is absorbed, phagocytized, presented to the lymph nodes, and then used for antibody production. Vaccination by injection (subcutaneous or intramuscular) stimulates the humoral immune system, requiring more time for antibody production.

How immune function is compromised

All animals are born with varying levels of natural resistance to foreign compounds, proteins, or infectious organisms or invaders. This is specific and different with each individual and different with each challenge. This can be physical (such as thicker hide or skin with certain breeds of cattle) to physiological differences with metabolism and ability to respond to stress or disease.

Primary genetic immune disorders do exist, and if sire changes have been made recently, it is necessary to consider genetic disorders for identifying the initial problem. The immune system is complex, and common disease problems can be caused by genetic weaknesses or susceptibility.

Primary immune system problems are those that originate at birth, while secondary immune system problems are due to immune depression caused by viruses, bacteria, toxins, cortisol from stress, or misuse of modified live virus (MLV) vaccine products causing immune suppression (temporary or permanent).

Breed influences can predispose calves to specific primary immune system problems related to the destruction and phagocytosis (sequestering) of bacteria by the immune system, as well as problems related to deficiencies in chemokines and cytokines that influence white blood cell (WBC) migration to the source of infection.

There exists a complex interaction between the immune system, stress, and nutrition.

Stress

Stress has a significant impact on immune system function, as cortisol produced by the adrenal cortex of a stressed animal *directly in-*

hibits normal immune function, both cellular and humoral. Even with good management and nutrition, stress can have disastrous effects on health. Stress can be manifested as dust, heat, cold, wetness, wind, crowding, human interaction, other animal interactions, and normal processing such as vaccination. Any novel or rare experience for an animal can be a source of stress causing physiological and psychological changes in the animal.

The best ranchers that have good economical results are often the ranches that have the lowest stress levels on cattle. Ranchers that have added reduced-stress handling to the ranch management decisions have experienced economic gains. Disposition is a key factor in stress, as seen with results in feedlot performance, as docile calves outperform calves that are restless or aggressive. This factor will be more important as economic pressures dictate purchase factors toward calves with quieter disposition traits.

Stress during transport has an important effect on performance after arrival. Key factors influencing level of transport stress include pre-transport management, noise, vibration, novelty, social regrouping, crowding, temperature, humidity, restraint, feed and water deprivation, and time of transit. Fear is also an important psychological stressor during handling and transport of cattle. Previous experience with handling and transport as well as genetic composition determines level of fear response of the animal.[70]

Stress during transport and marketing can compromise the immune system and predisposes cattle to develop certain infectious diseases, including the bovine respiratory disease (BRD) complex.[71] Humoral

---

70. Grandlin, 1997.
71. Dubeski et al., 1996.

immune response is decreased by stresses of transportation and remains suppressed for several weeks.[72] When combined with abrupt weaning prior to transportation, the effect on humoral immunity is additive.[73]

The most critical factor in transit stress is time in transit. The following table estimates shrink with respect to time.

Hours in truck	Percent shrink	Days to recover weight
1 hr.	2%	0
2–8 hrs.	2–4%	4–8
8–16 hrs.	5–6%	8–16
16–24 hrs.	8–10%	16–24
24–32 hrs.	10+%	24–30

Table 12: *Relationship of % shrink to hours of transport in a truck.*[74]

Upon arrival, changes in environment, complicated stress factors, and cattle handling management often lead to calves not eating. It has been reported that as many as 67% percent of received calves are not on full feed for three days after arrival.[75] This nutritional deprivation drastically affects immune response and predisposes the calves to disease.

Another widely accepted stressor of beef cattle is commingling. When calves from various sources are commingled in feedlot pens, the social hierarchy is destroyed, and additional stress is imposed.[76]

72. McKenzie et al., 1997.
73. Mckenzie et al., 1997; Pollard et al., 1997.
74. Fox et al., 1985.
75. Smith, 2005, Sager, 2012.
76. Loerch and Fluharty, 2000.

If the calf becomes sick, energy resources are re-directed to support an immune response, which means that energy is not available for growth.

Nutrition

The following diagram shows the relation of mineral deficiency to body function. The first function to decrease due to mineral deficiencies is the immune system, before growth and performance. This concept is poorly understood, and the immediate signs are hidden from the producer as immune system function can't be measured or evaluated by quantitative means in the same way as most other performance measures.

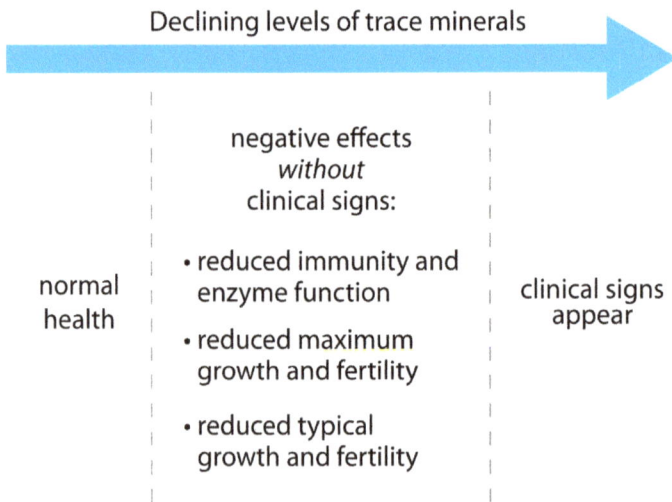

Declining levels of trace minerals

negative effects
without
clinical signs:

normal
health

• reduced immunity and
  enzyme function

• reduced maximum
  growth and fertility

• reduced typical
  growth and fertility

clinical signs
appear

Figure 15: *Effects of reduced trace mineral status. Negative effects occur before clinical signs appear.*[77]

The ultimate economic goal in beef cattle production is the achieve-

77. *Montana State University handout, Bozeman, MT.*

ment of a high percentage calf crop each year, as most beef cattle producers are interested in the most economical return per cow bred the year before. No area of beef cattle production is as essential to reaching that goal as nutrition. To get a return, the heifer or cow must be bred. This involves many physiological or biological factors, all directly and strongly influenced by nutritional intake, absorption, and utilization of nutrients. Nutrition influences net return, and cows gaining positive body weight before breeding show faster estrus return, higher conception, and higher pregnancy maintenance.

Calf crop return is most influenced by the period 60 days before breeding and the first 60–70 post-breeding; a period of less than one third of the year but highly critical. This period sets up the rest of the calving year, as the cow is lactating, growing a fetus, and still trying to maintain or increase BCS. Differences vary between breeds and frame size, but the following is a guide or suggestion for nutrient requirements of breeding beef cows.

The impact of nutrition: A case report

During 2001 and 2002 several vaccine-failure problems in nursing beef calves initiated diagnostic investigation to determine causes of BRD in four-month-old calves. Confirmation of primary copper (Cu) deficiency causing failure of normal immune response was determined with liver biopsy analysis. Copper deficiency was determined to be a result of antagonistic interactions with iron (Fe), molybdenum (Mo), and sulfates (SO_4). Geological soil analysis showed a Mo:Cu ratio of 8:1. Iron in the soil and water was several times higher than recommended levels. Sulfate levels were 3 times higher than previous analysis due to 6-to-7 years of draught.

BRD signs decreased within 1-week after $CuSO_4$ supplementation in water tanks at a dosage of 300 ppm for 10 days and 150 ppm for another 30 days. Bovine respiratory disease decreased and calves grew at a normal rate until weaning in October. Weaning weights were 97% of normal, and BRD during the feeding period was normal compared to past years.

Changing nutritional requirements

In the past 50 years, United States beef cattle production has increased nearly 50% due to improved genetics, advances in nutrition, bio-technology, advances in animal health, and value-added management.[78] Much of this is due to a better understanding of nutrition related to health.

The National Research Council (NRC) requirements for beef cattle were first published in the 1950's when production requirements for beef cattle production were two-thirds of present day production expectations.[79] Recommended NRC levels were derived from experiments during the 1950's using cattle that were genetically different, raised with a different production focus, and fed different diets. Today beef cattle production involves animals that are 35–40% larger anatomically, grow at increased rates, and are developed with more focus on muscle growth with efficient gain than 50 years ago.

Beef cattle are now grown in larger feeding facilities with increased population densities and increased microbial environments that potentially magnify pathogen densities and increased risk for BRD. Modern beef cattle feedlots do increase efficiency of production, but inadvertently cause increases in BRD.

---

78. Paterson, 2010

79. NRC, 2005.

Since these factors have all changed, requirements for all minerals and vitamins in beef cattle production have likely increased. Large-scale production units now use customized mineral programs based on water and forage analysis compared to requirements for the age, desired growth goals, and gestational requirements of the animals being fed.

Mineral and Vitamin Deficiencies

There are many nutritional factors that dramatically affect the immune system, but *none are more common than protein and energy deficiencies.* The next-most-common are mineral and vitamin deficiencies, which are just as serious, but harder to diagnose. Minerals most often seen as problems are Selenium (Se), Copper (Cu), Manganese (Mn), Cobalt (Co), and Zinc (Zn).

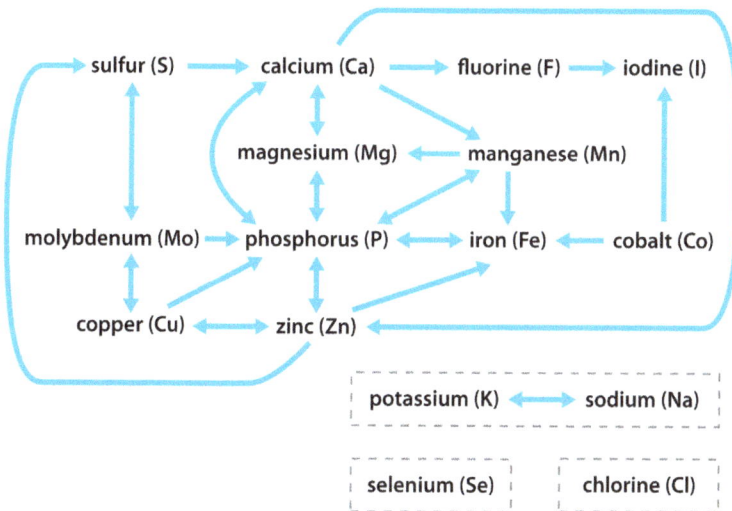

Figure 16: *Potential antagonism between minerals. The interactions between minerals are complex.*

These minerals are often provided in recommended or required National Research Council levels, but the calf remains deficient due to antagonistic interference from plant, soil, or water components. Water and forage analysis need to be completed on a regular and timely basis to minimize nutritional problems from antagonistic interference.

These problems are highly complex and require detailed analysis and professional help so that corrective management decisions can be made. One must remember the calf is often marginal or deficient in body nutrients and immune system function at birth, because it has developed from nutrients taken from the dam during gestation.

Also, although milk is nature's ideal food, it is not fortified with the specific vitamins, minerals, or proteins necessary to endure added stress, infections, or for immediate recovery of deficiencies at birth. Colostrum is higher in immunoglobulins, protein, energy, and lactoferrins than milk obtained several days later. These components are necessary nutrients for life.

Trace mineral injections

Calves administered a trace mineral injection had reduced BRD compared with control calves. Administration of a trace mineral injection during initial processing of highly stressed, newly received heifers improved average daily gain, feed efficiency, BRD, and antibiotic treatment cost. Antibiotic treatment cost was greater for control calves than for calves treated with trace mineral injections at arrival to a feedlot.[80]

In another study completed at Oklahoma State University, an injectable trace mineral solution (Multimin) increased feed intake after

---

80. Richeson and Kegley, 2011.

arrival and increased average daily gain during the feeding period

The reduction in antibiotic treatment cost exceeded the cost of administering either of these injectable trace mineral solutions during processing. The cost of the mineral solution was less than $1.50 per animal.[81]

Preconditioning programs

Nutritional supplementation pre-weaning, without the need to rely on normal intake after arrival, needs to be considered. In recent years, preconditioning programs have added value for beef calf producers to establish marketing advantages and increased return profit from management decisions to immunize before weaning and shipment.

Preconditioning programs are designed to reduce stress associated with weaning, enhance the immune systems of calves, and teach calves to eat from a feed bunk and drink from a fountain or trough while remaining at their birth location for a 30-to-45-day post-weaning period.

Benefits of preconditioning to stocker and feedlot operators are well-established with less morbidity and mortality, improved post-weaning performance, and higher carcass quality. However, approximately 50% of calves sold at weaning do not have any preconditioning program in place.

Nutritional supplementation at pre-weaning has shown advantages post-weaning.[82] Calves from a single source that are retained on the ranch for 45 days after weaning exhibit less morbidity and less health costs during the receiving period at the feedlot than when cattle are

81. Richeson and Kegley, 2011.
82. Smith, 2005; Taylor, 2010.

commingled or trucked to the feedlot immediately after weaning.[83]

Vaccination

Cost and return-on-investment of vaccination

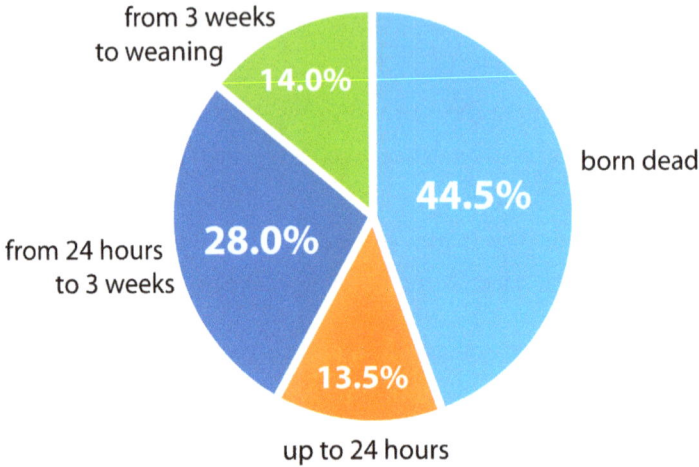

Figure 17: Percentage of calf deaths by age at death, for the first 6 months of life.[84]

Calves lost before weaning are a major cost in ranch operations, and the graph above shows that losses at birth account for almost 50% of the total losses before weaning. Less than 14% of the total losses occur after 3 weeks after birth. This reflects the proper use of vaccination before and at branding to minimize death losses.

Clostridial infections have almost been eliminated thanks to nearly 100% use of multiple Clostridial vaccines in beef calves, along with the use of viral respiratory vaccine combinations which have mini-

83. Step et al., 2008.

84. Data adapted from figures provided by USDA-NAHMS, 2008.

mized summer pneumonia.

The past two decades have introduced pre-weaning programs for specific marketing to direct buyers who only purchase calves from certified vaccination programs. This has led to increased value through weaned calves having fewer health problems on arrival at feedlots, and has added trust and profit through calves purchased by repeat buyers.

Data supports the idea that calves from non-pre-weaned vaccination programs are twenty times more likely to get pneumonia when shipped to a feedlot than immunized calves.[85]

In the feedlot, one time through the chute is considered equal to a seven-day feeding period.[86] The producer should focus on four areas of health performance for maximizing performance after the calf is weaned. These include:

+ Pre-weaning vaccination

+ Stress reduction

+ Resolving or improving nutritional concerns pre-weaning

+ Reducing parasite problems

Recent vac-like programs have proven cost-effective, have added trust and profit with buyers, and have added value to beef calf operations. For vaccination costs of $2.00–3.75 per calf (depending on products required by specific programs), and with added labor, programs are still profitable for producers and increase probability of repeat buyers and possible increased returns the next year based

85. Whittier, et al., 2000.

86. Whittier, et al., 2000.

on health performance at the feedlot.

It has been estimated that the time spent in pre-weaning immunization is worth more than $1000 per hour in preventing post-weaning problems. Pre-conditioning is cost-effective, adds value to the calf, and is highly effective in promotion of calf welfare and health.

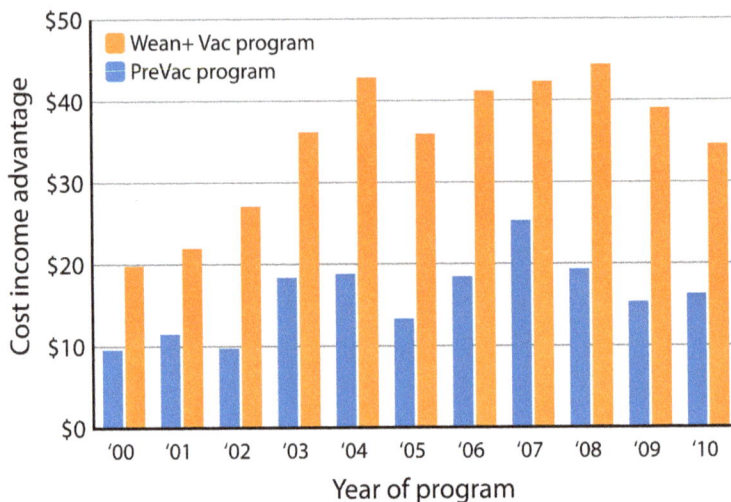

Figure 18: *Price differential for vaccination programs, for a 540 lb. calf, comparison of two programs versus no program.*[87]

A 10-year average of pre-vac calves was over $17.00 more profitable per calf than non-vac calves, representing *over a $1700.00 increase per 100 calves at weaning.*

Decreased sickness and improved health at the feedlot results in improved carcass quality and higher yield.[88] For each time an animal is treated in the feedlot, a loss of $85.20 is incurred (see following table).

87. Chart taken from Pfizer Animal Health vaccination program handout.

88. Smith, 2005.

# of sick treatments	0	1	2
Avg. daily gain	3.2 lbs.	3.0 lbs.	2.9 lbs.
Mortality rate	0.10%	0.13%	10.00%
Grade Choice and Choice+	74.3%	64.7%	57.6%
Grade Standard	2.2%	4.9%	9.3%
Treatment costs	(par)	-$20.60	-$48.43
Avg. daily gain *	(par)	-$24.49	-$35.71
Death loss discount	(par)	-$31.07	-$100.04
Carcass weight discount	(par)	-$1.56	-$1.58
Dark cutter discount	(par)	+$0.18	-$0.58
Quality grade premium	(par)	-$10.39	-$19.41
Yield grade premium	(par)	+$2.90	+$4.59
Net return	(par)	-$85.03	-$201.16

* Avg. daily gain based on lbs of additional carcass weight gained during feeding period.

Table 13: *Effect of post-weaning disease on performance, carcass, and profitability.*[89]

The preceding data comes from a certified Angus Beef and Iowa State University study that was completed on over 13,321 calves from 12 states fed in 8 Iowa feedlots from 2002–2004.

From this data, post-weaning sickness had significant impact on feedlot gain, carcass characteristics and performance, mortality rate, treatment costs, and profit. Some have commented that all that are

89. Data from Paterson, 2009, *Beef / Cattle Extension Program, What are the Effects of Calf Health on Feedlot Performance.* Original source: *Beef Cattle Research Update;* Michigan State University

involved in these programs profit and the quality of beef calf production is increased. These programs are observed by the end consumers as added welfare applied to the beef cattle industry and can be perceived as added value in product purchases.

In this study the disposition of the calf was correlated with performance. Docile calves returned $13.13 more than restless calves at harvest, and $62.19 more than aggressive calves. The combination of post-weaning sickness and disposition have a huge additional negative influence on feedlot performance and profits. Break-even costs are used to assess feedlot performance by many feedlot consultants. The table below uses a natural raised steer model assuming an average daily gain of 2.87 lb. (1.3 kg) and a gain per unit of feed (G:F) of 0.14.

Variable in economic model	Assumption (US $)
Incoming body weight (BW)	550 lbs.
Laid-in price	$1.10/lb.
Vaccination costs	$2.50
De-wormer costs	$1.60
Feed cost	$171.00/ton
Days on feed	210
Yardage per day	$0.30/head/day
Interest rate	6.5%
Outgoing body weight (BW)	1252 lbs.
Shrink	4.00%
Fat cattle price	$0.96

Table 14: The estimated break-even costs for natural feedlot performance. (Data from 2010.)

Vaccination guidelines and recommendations

Much consideration should be used in deciding between modified live virus (MLV) and killed vaccine, and producers should be advised by an expert or local veterinarian that knows your herd health needs, ranch production goals, and yearly management decisions. Designing a vaccination program for a specific ranch or client requires a knowledge of the ranch's history and a basic understanding of vaccine immunology. There is no better person to have the history and basic science than the ranch's veterinarian. Products chosen should meet the specific needs of the ranch first and have efficacy for producing the desired result. The adaption of ranch management procedures should also be considered in terms of when the animals needing vaccination will be accessible to handle and work.

Each program offers specific advantages and disadvantages. Briefly, MLV vaccines have advantages in that the vaccine products mimic natural disease organisms that are recognized by the immune system as natural pathogens, and therefore give a more specific response. Generally, these products produce a longer-lasting immunity, and because they are "live", replicate in the body and stimulate a higher level of response. They do not contain endotoxins (unlike killed products), and do not require boosters to be given 3–4 weeks apart. Also, MLV products generally have costs that are lower for the same antigenic products than killed products. Care and handling recommendations should be strictly adhered to in using all products. Care should be used in keeping products cool, and not mixing MLV products more than one hour before use. Products should be kept out of sunlight and protected from freezing in cold weather. Read labels carefully, and if you have questions, call the listed numbers (provided on the labeling or outside the box of the product) or your animal health provider. Much technical support is provided by animal health companies for your information. If you cannot contact your veterinarian or animal health provider, use the web site or telephone numbers provided. Always check before choosing and using products.

Vaccination Schedule for calves

Vaccine	Recommended?	Age of immunization
Blackleg 7-Way	yes	Branding and pre-weaning
IBR-BVD-PI3	yes	Branding and pre-weaning
Leptospirosis	yes	Consult local vet
Brucellosis	yes	Replacement heifers (4–12 months)
BRSV	yes	Branding and pre-weaning
Pasteurella	yes	Branding and pre-weaning
Histophilus or Haemophilus somnus	yes	Consult local vet
Pinkeye	optional	As needed
E. coli	optional	Vaccinate cows (twice first year) 30 days before calving
Anthrax	optional	Consult local vet
Anaplasmosis	optional	Consult local vet

Table 15: List of commonly recommended vaccination products for beef calf production.

Metaphylaxis

A popular method of minimizing sickness on feedlot calves upon arrival is to mass treat all calves with injectable antibiotics (an approach known as metaphylaxis). Newer, long-lasting antibiotics (Micotil, Draxxin, or Nuflor) are popular products that minimize sickness, decrease morbidity, and decrease days of treatment and off-feed days, allowing for a faster start in average daily gain and carcass quality. These products are approximately $4.05-$18.15 per head depending on the product used. These values offset the initial costs, but for high-risk calves this has proven to have economic value. Cattle that were treated and received a metaphylaxis on arrival showed an increased average daily gain of 0.24lb (0.1kg) per day, compared to those that did not receive treatment.

The value of the cattle (not a risk factor, but important in the decision to use metaphylaxis) is often considered for metaphylaxis recommendation. Risk factors important for decision making usually include the following, although every situation is different:

+ Vaccination and de-worming history of cattle is the most important.

+ Commingled vs. single-source cattle. Commingled calves are at a much higher risk for sickness than single-source calves.

+ Age of the calves (older is riskier), and body size of the cattle (smaller, lighter-weight calves are more susceptible).

+ Sex of the cattle (bulls are considered higher risk than steers).

+ Time of the year (spring vs. fall), which usually involves a consideration of weather factors.

+ Weaned vs. un-weaned (un-weaned calves are more prone to sickness, as the stress is a key factor in reducing feed intake and lowers natural immune system functions).

+ The operator's ability to detect and treat sick calves (facilities are very important)

+ Previous problems or history of Bovine Respiratory Disease (BRD) problems

Typically, a decision to consider mass treatment of the next arrival is based on a 10% threshold: if 10% of the calves are treated for three consecutive days, then mass treatment is recommended.

The use of implants increased average daily gain in steers by 0.55 lbs. (0.25kg) per day, increased feed consumption dry matter intake (DMI) by 1.17 lb, and improved gain per unit of feed (G:F) by 0.02 (P<0.01).[90]

These improved performance gains are the result of the use of new technology in increasing beef production efficiency, with results that increase profit. A return on investment as high as 8–20 times costs can be realized using implants and other newer technology. These most often also result in decreasing ecological concerns and are environmentally sound.

Modified live virus (MLV) vs. killed

A discussion of these terms could result in many pages of explanation. The bottom line is that *you should discuss the positives and negatives with your local animal health professional or veterinarian.* Generally, it is best to be on an MLV program, because of advantages in immune system response, economical cost of product and handling, and length of protection. One of the best advantages is that *MLV vaccines mimic the natural disease stimulation of the immune system, and MLV units reproduce and stimulate immune response better.*

Generally, killed vaccines require two separate doses given 2–4 weeks apart for best response, and are usually more expensive. However,

---

90. Wileman and Thomson, 2010.

killed vaccines do have advantages in some cases over MLV products. *One potential problem is endotoxin mass and the need for better
storage and protection. Freezing of killed vaccines can cause endotoxins
to be released in the product, which can cause anaphylactic shock and
possible death when used later.*

A note on genetic engineering and immunity

It is thought by knowledgeable professionals that through the over
fifty years of selection for genetic traits for growth, muscling, milk
production, and through a lack of heterozygous breeding, that we
have inadvertently developed a genetic tendency for increased problems with disease, metabolic problems, and loss of resistance to common infection, parasitism, and natural selection physiology.

In my career I have personally seen increased incidence of pneumonias, an increase in abomasal ulcers, and increased incidence of
enteric Clostridia infections such as Clostridium perfringens type
C and A. I do not personally believe it is all due to increased production and metabolic and physiological stress. This problem area
needs to be explored more. Genetic engineering is pioneering traits
for resistance to disease. Great interest in this area is getting much
attention at present time.

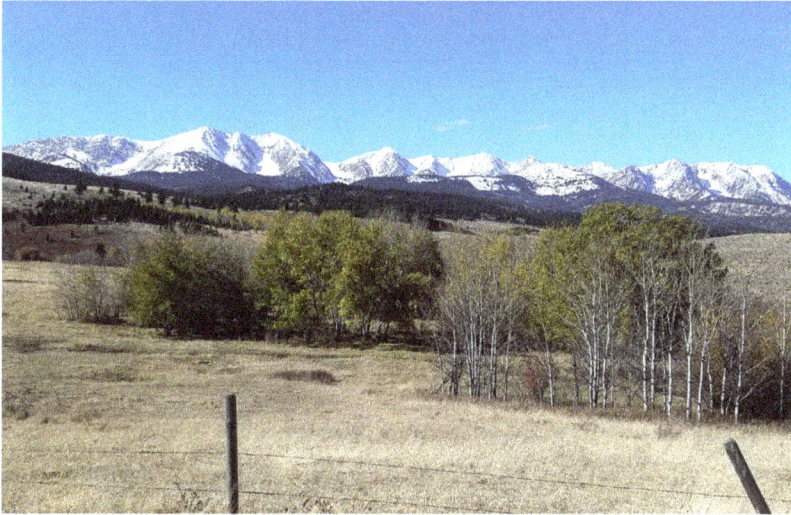

6

Necropsy of the Beef Calf

The basic calf necropsy, also commonly called a post-mortem exam, is an examination of an animal after death. The main objective is to obtain an accurate cause of death.

This chapter will give you the knowledge necessary to identify the obvious visual symptoms of common calf diseases, and to obtain tissue samples that will allow for a full clinical analysis that will proceed to a definitive diagnosis. With determined practice, you can become proficient at performing a basic field necropsy, which can help to prevent losses in your herd by identifying certain diseases as soon as possible. However, please keep the following two warnings in mind at all times.

Warning: This chapter is not a substitute for the advice of a veterinarian or another professional.

Performing your own field necropsy can save crucial time and money. However, if you try to substitute yourself for a veterinarian, it will ultimately cost you time, money, and risk the safety of you and your herd. Do not overreach your own abilities.

Warning: Be alert for any possibility of zoonotic diseases (those which can transfer from animals to humans). Carefully read all the warnings in this chapter about zoonotics.

Do not risk infecting yourself under any circumstances, and do not proceed with a necropsy if you become aware of the possibility of a zoonotic disease.

Overview

When performing a necropsy, the most important consideration is to look at the animal as a whole, as well as looking at each individual organ within the body. Deliberate and careful examination, with timely sampling of diseased organs, can help determine the cause of death, be it disease or trauma.

Warning: Be extremely careful when investigating a sudden death next to a water system that is supplied by an electrical pump, or near any electrical supply.

Often in these situations, electrocution is the cause of death. The animal may still be a source of electrical current and is therefore potentially lethal to you.

(Many times, animals will lick or chew on electrical wiring, or rub on insulators and other electrical supply items, causing an electrical contact. This is particularly common with electrical pumps that feed water tanks and waterers. Preventive measures to keep electrical components away from animals can reduce this type of death.)

Reasons for a necropsy

Some possible reasons for a necropsy include:

+ Identifying a cause of death so you can minimize future disease, or to identify appropriate treatments for the other animals in your herd.

+ Identifying the specific cause of death, so you can evaluate a potential change in vaccination programs, change of management techniques, or to help your understanding of the cause of the death.

+ Promotion of your calf health programs with your veterinarian or your animal health specialist.

+ Identification of a disease to determine whether it is zoonotic. (Zoonotics can be transferred to you, your workers, and your family.)

A crucial first consideration

Since the original shape and size of the animal carcass will be destroyed by the necropsy, it is ideal to take a digital picture before starting. Modern cell phone cameras have very good resolution and can be a good record source later if needed.

+ Record the animal's ID number, sex, breed, age in months, date, time, weather, and as many other factors as possible that can be recorded at the time of the necropsy. (Were there any visual signs prior to death? Any history of trauma or disease? Any other information that would be of value in determining the cause of death?)

+ Note where the animal died. Is there any evidence of the soil being disturbed, as in a struggle before death? Is there evidence of any activity before death? Were the animals near any metal, such as a metal wire fence with wood posts, instead of metal posts that would ground any possible lightning strike? (Was there an electrical storm in the past twenty-four hours?)

+ Consider a feed analysis if you suspect nutritional problems. Nutritional problems would almost always affect more than one animal, unless poisonous plants are a possibility (typically in early spring or during droughts). The "green plants" that emerge during early spring can entice calves to chew and consume a poisonous plant (even if there is still snow on the ground).

+ It's also best to take pictures of your findings before and during the necropsy, to show your veterinarian later.

Time necessary for an accurate diagnosis

Time of the necropsy is critical, especially in warm weather, as tissue changes occur rapidly and often within 20–30 minutes after death. Performing a necropsy at too late a time will make the necropsy worthless for identification of a specific cause of death or disease. Performing the necropsy promptly will allow tissue samples to provide an accurate diagnosis. Also note that the tissues of a febrile (fevered) animal will typically decompose much faster than in an animal that died from trauma.

Site Selection

Biosecurity is one of the most important considerations on determination of the necropsy site.

The necropsy should be performed in an area where there is no risk of spreading the disease to other herd animals.

+ Choose an area that can be easily and thoroughly disinfected.

+ Choose an area that is away from all high-traffic areas on the property, as well as away from any family activities.

+ Choose an area that is protected against any neighbor animals (such as dogs or cats) or local carnivores, either of which may scavenge tissues or the carcass, creating a threat of disease spread.

+ A concrete pad is ideal, but these are often located near high-traffic areas. For larger producers, a common "bone pile" is ideal, so carcasses can be buried later.

+ Most areas do not have a rendering service available, so the need to bury the carcass (if local laws allow) must be considered before the necropsy is started.

Supplies and equipment

Prepare the following equipment and supplies in advance:

+ A large pen or marker that can write on wet material (black marker works well).

+ Ziploc bags (at least 6), at least two sizes, with the larger at least 1qt. You will be labelling these bags.

- Large-mouthed plastic vials.

- Larger vials or jars.

- String or twine for tying off intestine samples

- Heavy packing tape

- Gloves, preferably latex, disposable (nitrile blue are stronger and recommended)

- Boots, rubber or plastic, that can be disinfected and washed thoroughly afterwards

- Protective plastic glasses

- Coveralls: disposable, or plastic or cloth that can be washed in disinfectant

- Two Boning knifes, 6". Most hunting knives will work well (not your wife's best carving knife).

- Steel, for sharpening the knife while completing the necropsy

- Large tree pruning shears, AKA rib cutters (or you can use an Ax)

- A bone saw or an ax for getting into the skull, and a large hammer for punching the ax blade through the skull bones.

- Disinfectant (chlorhexidine is a good standard disinfectant for this purpose).

Position of the calf

Usually it is best to start the necropsy with the calf laying on its left side (right side facing up). With calves older than 3 months, this allows for better exposure of the abdominal organs, both to be seen and for tissue samples to be taken. With age, the rumen becomes larger, and at six months and later occupies approximately one-half of the abdominal cavity. The size and weight of the rumen and contents makes it hard to move or remove when attempting to get samples of the liver and other organs, which are commonly needed for a definitive diagnosis. Furthermore, the liver is mostly on the right side, so facing the right side up makes it easier to recover liver tissues for a detailed mineral analysis and lab analysis if you suspect a mineral deficiency is leading to decreased immune function.

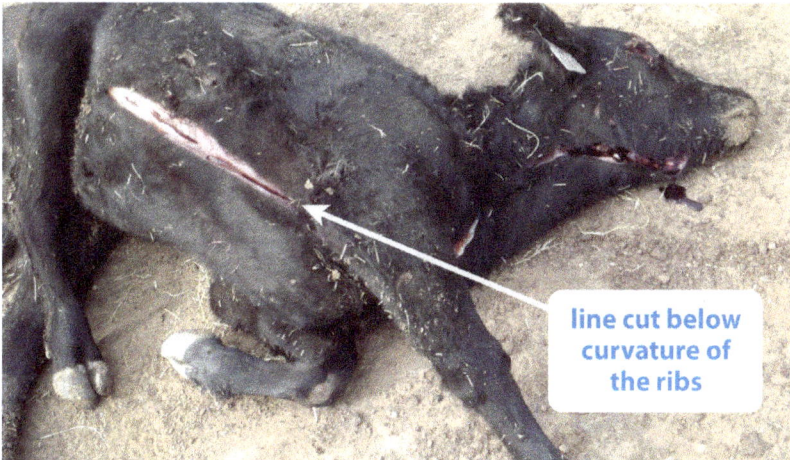

line cut below curvature of the ribs

Figure N1: *First incision.*

Inspection and First Incision

First, carefully inspect the entire animal, identify any signs of trauma, and note any obvious visual abnormalities. Bloody discharges from the nose, mouth, rectum, or vulva are critical for identifying specific diseases.

Warning: If you see a bloody discharge that is not coagulated, immediately stop and call your veterinarian.

This may be a case of Anthrax (Anthrax bacillus), which is lethal to humans. Do not place yourself in a lethal situation.

The first incision should be made from the jaw area to the rectum if right-handed, or from the rectum to the jaw area if left-handed. (The rest of this section assumes you are right-handed and are starting at the jaw.) Make this incision *only ½-inch deep*, to avoid penetrating the stomach and its contents. See Figure N1 (previous page).

Always perform the incision carefully and always push the knife away from you. Don't pull the knife toward your body. As you perform more procedures, you will gain experience in knowing the proper depth of the incision.

Continue the skin incision along the body, between the legs, and above the mammary area and above the external genitalia (bull calf or steer calf).

Dissect the hide away from the ribcage and over the back, while cutting the underlying tissues. By dissecting and cutting away the connective tissue between the hide and the muscle and other connective tissues that are immediately below, you will make it possible to fold over the hide for exposure of the underlying carcass.

As you cut between the front legs, the front leg can be folded over the carcass toward the back. See Figure N2 (facing page). The hind leg can be lifted to cut into the hip joint and fold the hind leg backward. The hip joint has a solid round ligament that can be cut once you get into the joint capsule. Continue in cutting through this ligament to allow the joint to come apart from the underlying pelvic structures. Once you have completed this, the hind limb will lay at a right angle to the body of the animal.

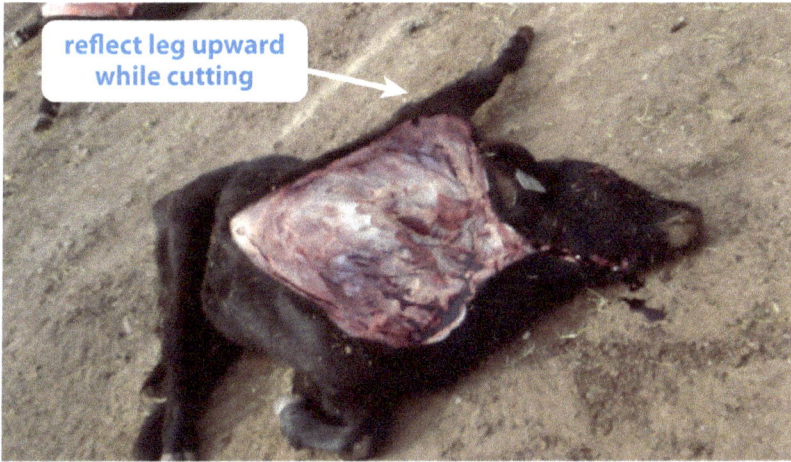

Figure N2: *Reflect leg upward.*

Once you have folded away the top front leg and top hind leg, you can finish exposing the thoracic and abdominal areas. Make a cut, parallel to the last rib and behind it, from the lowest point upward toward the back. See Figure N3 (next page). Once this cut is completed, use a steel or other metal instrument to pull the abdominal wall away from the internal organs as you cut the connective tissue. Be careful not to cut into the stomach and other organs.

Remember to cut away from your body and be careful at all times. Applying pressure against a morbid animal can cause a knife to slip very easily.

At this point you have access to the abdominal cavity to observe any abnormalities and collect any diseased tissues for analysis.

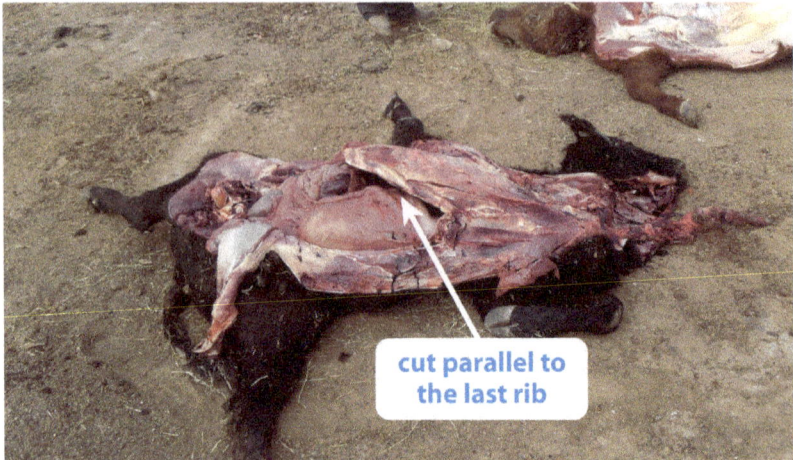

Figure N3: Cut parallel to last rib.

The next step is to extend the cut behind the rib cage to expose the thoracic cavity. Cut parallel to the back bone and reflect the muscles to expose the ribs.

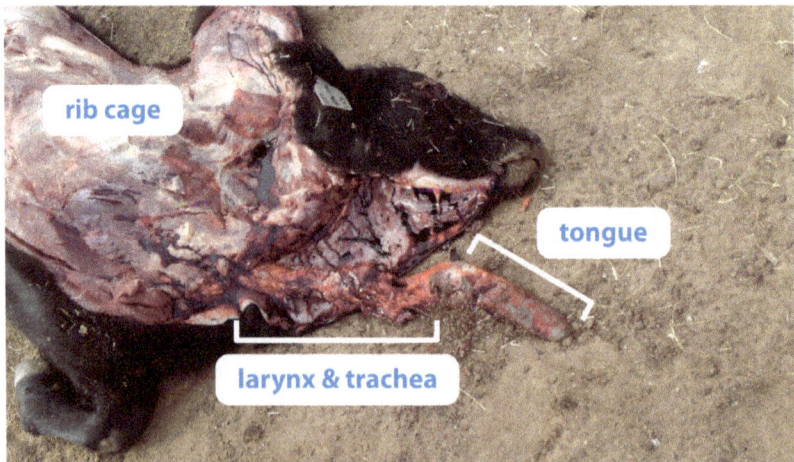

Figure N4: Rib cage, tongue, larynx, trachea.

Using a saw, cut through as many ribs as possible. Cut the sternum from the end toward the head. This allows the thoracic cavity to be exposed, showing the lungs and heart in the lower anterior portion of the cavity.

The jaw area between the jaw bones can be cut as a "V", starting from the front teeth area and cutting backwards along the sides of the jaw bones to expose the tongue. Continue downward to the neck area, exposing the trachea. This entire section can be removed outside the carcass by cutting at the thoracic inlet at the beginning of the rib cage. See Figure N4 (facing page).

In calves under 8 months of age, approximately 50% or more of the pathology that leads to increased costs and calf deaths can be attributed to pulmonary problems (pneumonia and respiratory illness and related causes). This is especially true in "sudden death" cases, where acute pneumonia will cause lungs to fill with fluid, causing the calf to die due to asphyxiation.

You do not have to be experienced to detect diseased tissues. If the carcass is not spoiled, diseased tissues usually are markedly different in texture and color, and have fibrin (yellow protein material) attached. With more experience, you will become more skilled in recognizing diseased tissues.

Figures N5–N7 on the following pages show examination of the trachea, lungs, heart, rumen, and small intestine.

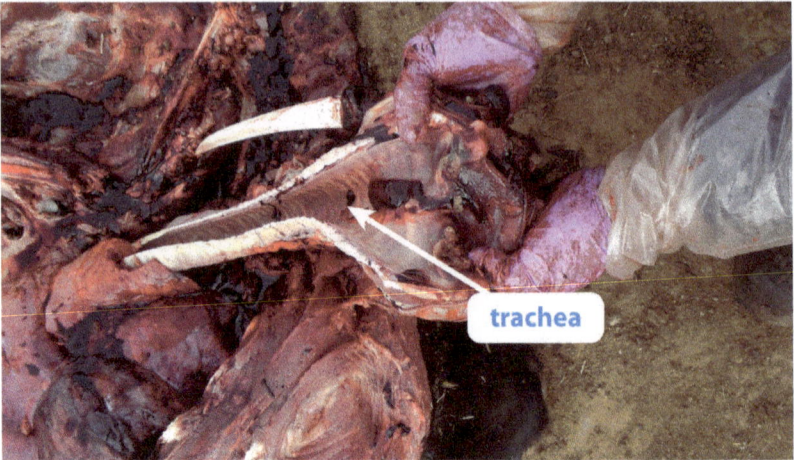

Figure N5: *Trachea.*

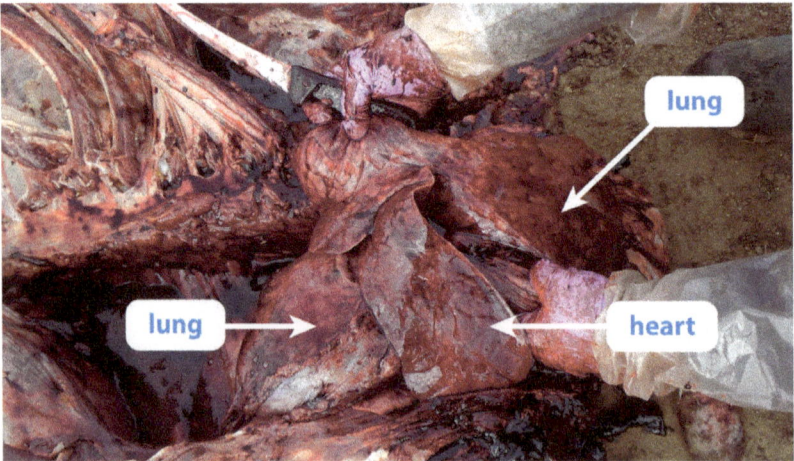

Figure N6: *Lungs and heart.*

The image above shows the heart and both lungs removed from the chest cavity for closer examination.

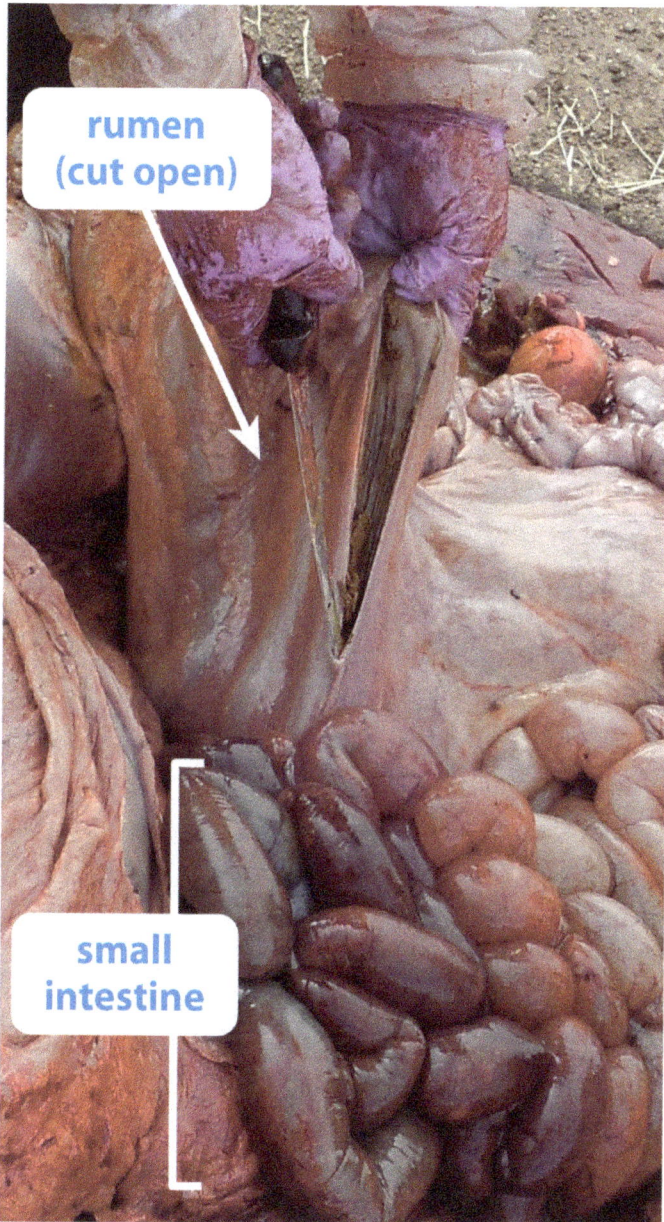

Figure N7: *Rumen cut open.*

Additional resources

There are excellent sources online to further develop your skills and knowledge:

+ https://www.cvmbs.colostate.edu/ilm/proinfo/necropsy/notes/Necropsy%20Manual.pdf

+ https://www.aphis.usda.gov/animal_health/lab_info_services/downloads/NecropsyGuideline.pdf

+ http://www.newportlabs.com/sites/newportlabs/files/NL4526%20Bovine%20Disease%20Manual.pdf

Transporting samples

+ When you collect samples for professional examination, each tissue needs to be preserved in a refrigerated or frozen state. Samples should be placed in a separate container—preferably plastic, not glass.

+ If you need to preserve tissues, the recommended preservative for tissue histological examination is 10% buffered neutral formalin. Formalin can be found at most pharmacies or at your veterinarian clinic. You may also be able to order it online.

+ Use separate pairs of latex gloves to collect the initial piece of each organ aseptically (without contamination) for microbiological examination. This is important to avoid contaminating samples.

+ Ensure that samples are kept moist, as drying of the sample will prevent further laboratory diagnosis.

+ Place any swabs in transport medium, or a sterile saline

solution in a small container or test tube.

+ Time is critical, so use overnight service preferably.

+ Samples of intestinal contents can be collected with a large needle and syringe and placed into a new container. Or, sections of the bowel can be tied off with string, twine, or rubber band, and sent refrigerated.

+ Samples of major organs and brain tissue should be completed by professionals, as cross sections will often interfere with a proper diagnosis. In addition, zoonotic viral diseases like Rabies can be transferred through aerosol drops or handling of infected tissues.

+ Experience will prove that the extra cost of overnight shipping is worthwhile for the increased accuracy of diagnosis. You have already spent the time and energy to go this far, so make sure that the shipment to the laboratory is the most efficient and timely one that you can make.

+ Try not to ship on a Thursday, as this can result in the samples sitting unrefrigerated over the weekend, especially in hot weather seasons. Even icing will not preserve samples for more than 48 hours in most cases. Proper preservation of samples is critical, as even the best lab and most skilled pathologists cannot salvage a ruined sample.

Conclusion

This chapter is not a complete reference on bovine necropsy. However, it has given you the basic information necessary to perform a field necropsy and to help identify common diseases and probable causes of death. It is important to work together with your veterinarian and laboratory personnel as much as possible. Over time, your increased knowledge and experience will help you take correct action in future cases, minimizing potential future problems in your operation.

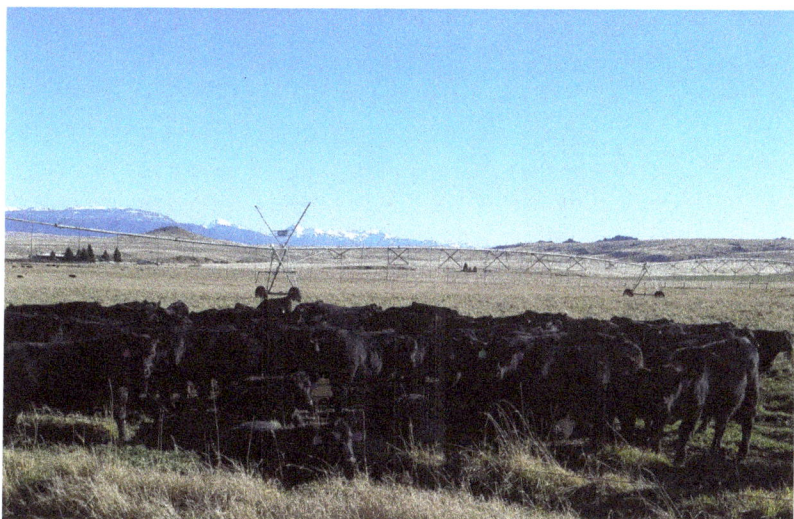

7

Common Products for Beef Calf Health

This chapter contains a review of common products used in the field, including purchasing information and advice for use.

Colostrum products

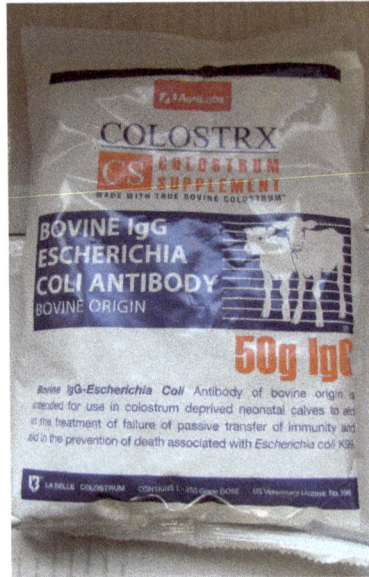

Image P06: *Colostrix Bovine IgG Antibody Powder*

©2016 AgriLabs
20927 State Hwy K
P.O. Box 3103 (64503)
(800) 542-8916
St Joseph, MO 64505

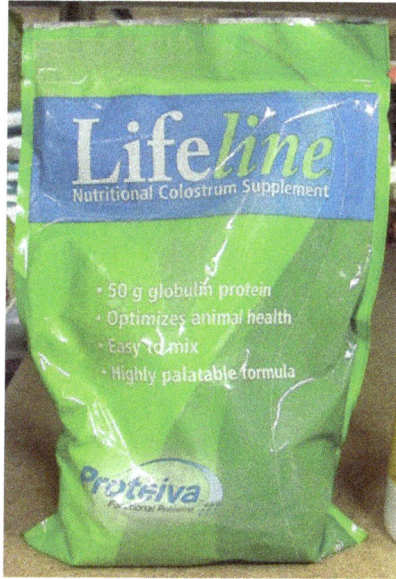

Image P01: *Commercial colostrum supplement.*

Most products contain >50 grams IgG—the more the better. Timing is the critical factor, rather than amount given. Multiple treatments are better than a single large-volume treatment. These are excellent products. Do not be microwave. For chilled calves, use warm water to increase body temperature.

Proteiva Functional Proteins
Proteiva, Ankeny, IA
info@proteiva.com

Electrolye products for oral fluid replacement

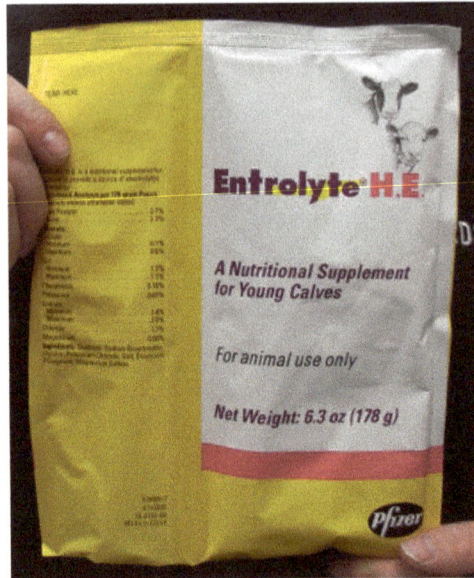

Image P03: *Commercial electrolyte supplement used for rehydrating calves with scour problems.*

Entrolyte H.E. by Pfizer Animal Health, www.pfizerah.com.

Most electrolytes have undergone decades of improvement and use. Remember it is the fluid or water that is the critical factor. Products will vary in their percentage of ingredients. Lifeguard HE has more energy and is a good value that has been proven through the years.

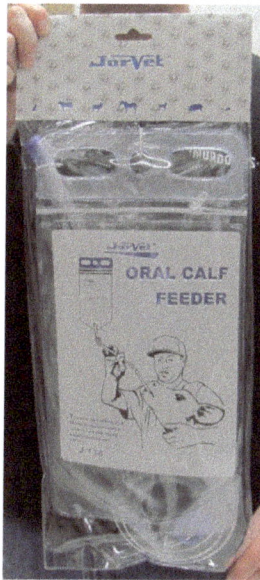

Image P02: *Calf feeder bag used for oral administration of fluids and electrolytes.*

Jorvet by Jorgenson
Loveland, CO
info@jorvet.com

Products for use in calf scours and pneumonia

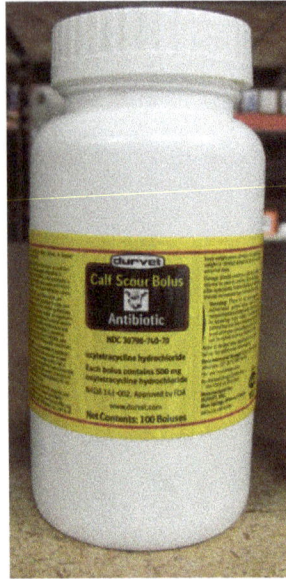

Image P07: *Durvet calf scour boluses (oral oxytetracycline tablets).*

The use of oral antibiotics has decreased greatly in the last twenty years. The protocol and recommendation of fluid therapy only with the use of probiotic products has shown better results.

I actually prefer no oral antibiotics, as these will upset normal flora that are of benefit to the calf. By comparison, oral fluids act to flush the entire GI tract of harmful toxins and bacteria.

Durvet Animal Health
Blue Springs, MO
www.durvet.com

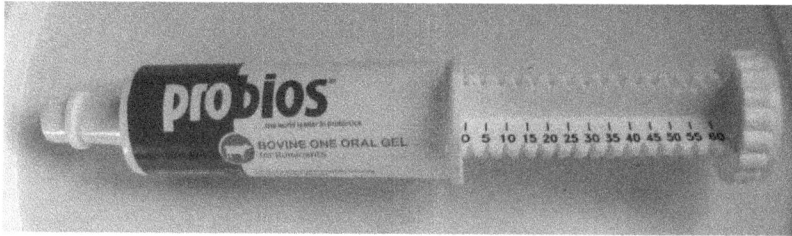

Image P08: *Probios oral gel. Replaces normal microflora. For use against pathogenic bacteria in the diarrhea calf.*

This is an excellent product to re-establish normal helpful bacteria and add energy and vitamins for calf health.

Includes added vitamins, natural vitamin E, over 1.5 billion colony-forming units (CFUs) of beneficial bacteria, plus Inulin, a food source for the bacteria.

Vets Plus, Inc. 302 Cedar Falls Road
Menomonie WI 54751
1-715-231-1235
http://www.Vets-Plus.com

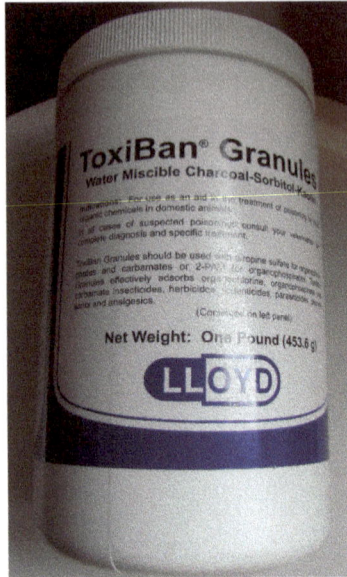

Image P09: *Toxiban, charcoal granules that absorb toxins.*

Toxiban is an activated charcoal product that does two things: absorb toxins form enteric bacteria that are harmful and depressive to the calf, and act as a marker so you can determine the GI passage rate of material. Toxiban is extremely messy, so use one fluid feeder bag for this product.

Lloyd Laboratories Inc.
#10 Lloyd Ave., FBIC
City of Malolos, Philippines
(+63-2) 411-5860 / 411-5884
(+63-2) 376-2284 / 376-2185
www.lloydlab.com

Injectable antibiotics

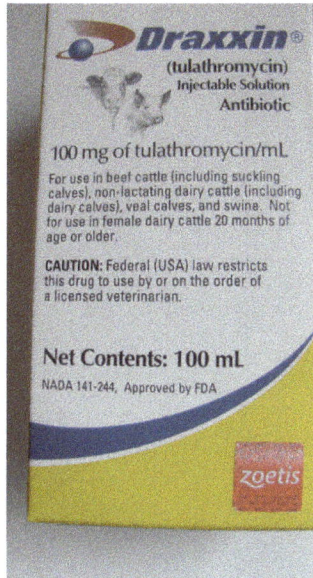

Images P10: *Draxxin, injectable tulathromycin.*

Draxxin is very good for young calf respiratory infections, and I have used this product with much success. It is "tissue-friendly", absorbed well, small dosage, and reaches lung tissues in 90 minutes for therapeutic action. It can be overused in some areas on calves that do not require it, and the product may show resistance in a few years.

Zoetis Animal Health
1-888-ZOETIS-1 (or 1-888-963-8471)

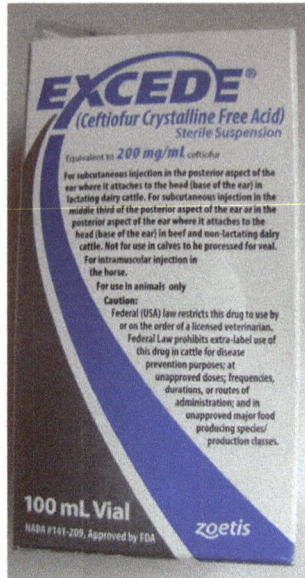

Images P11: *Excede, injectable ceftiofur.*

Zoetis Animal Health
1-888-ZOETIS-1 (or 1-888-963-8471)

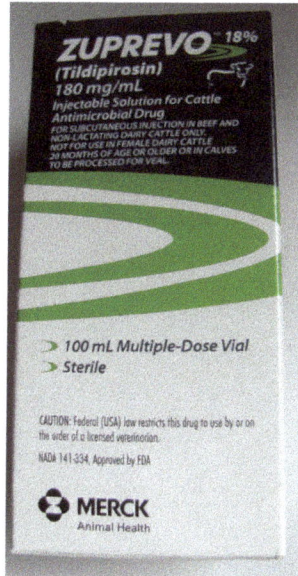

Image P12: Zuprevo, injectable florfenicol.

Merck Animal Health U.S. Corporate Headquarters
2 Giralda Farms
Madison, NJ 07940
animal-health-communications@merck.com

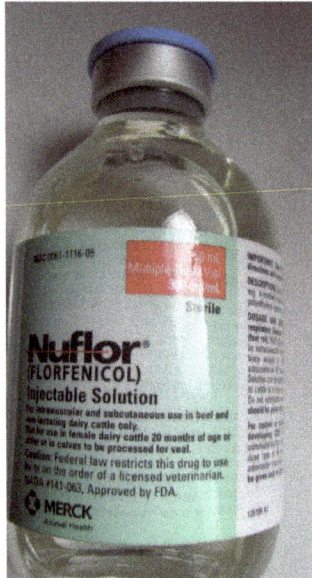

Images P13: *Nuflor, injectable florfenicol.*

Merck Animal Health
U.S. Corporate Headquarters
2 Giralda Farms
Madison, NJ 07940
animal-health-communications@merck.com

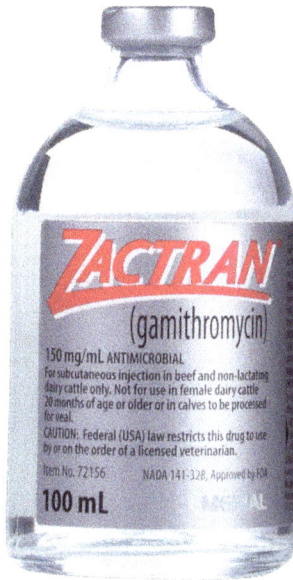

Image P14: *Zactran, injectable gamithromycin.*

Zactran, like Zuprevo, is one of the newer antibacterial products that can be used successfully for BRD. I have used these products in larger calves because of the small dosage and effectiveness.

Merial Limited
3239 Satellite Blvd #500
Duluth, GA 30096 USA
+1 678 638 3000

Other commonly-used products

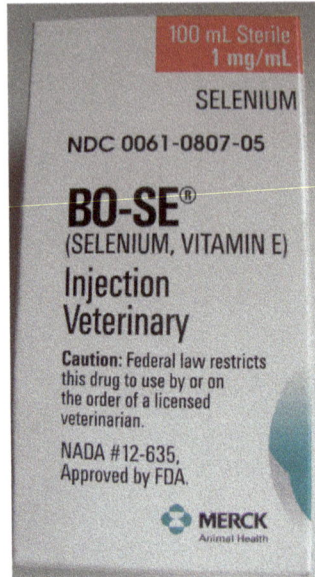

Image P15: *Bo-Se, injectable Selenium and Vitamin E.*

Merck Animal Health U.S. Corporate Headquarters
2 Giralda Farms
Madison, NJ 07940
animal-health-communications@merck.com

Used for stimulating the calf immune system and for prevention of White Muscle Disease. Use of this product in Se-marginal or Se-deficienct areas is one of the most effective management decisions you can make when tagging calves at birth. I had a rancher in my practice use it on every other calf, and the treated calves were 15 pounds heavier at weaning than the calves that did not receive the product. Excellent value; oil-based product lasts for weeks.

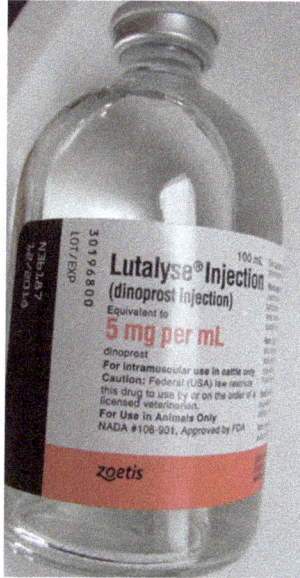

Image P16: *Lutylase. Dinoprost injectable, 5mg/mL.*

1-888-ZOETIS-1 (or 1-888-963-8471)

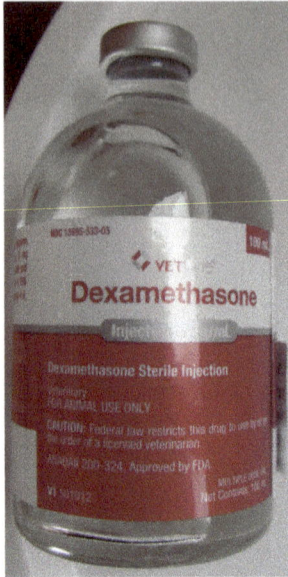

Image P17: *Dexamethasone (synthetic dexamethasone injectable). Injectable corticosteroid for anti-inflammatory use.*

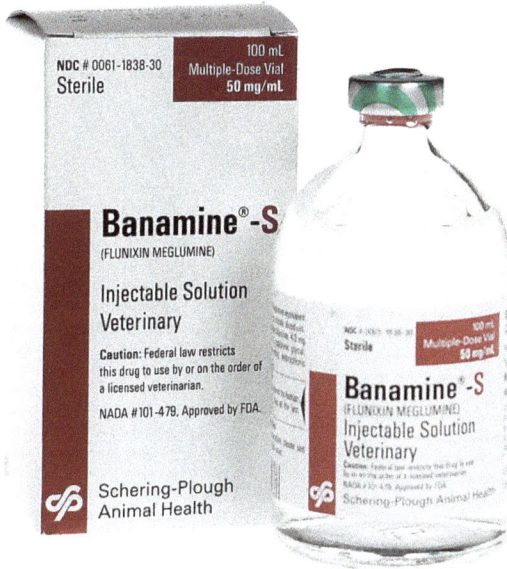

Image P18: *Banamine, injectable anti-inflammatory.*

Merck Animal Health U.S. Corporate headquarters
2 Giralda Farms
Madison, NJ 07940
animal-health-communications@merck.com

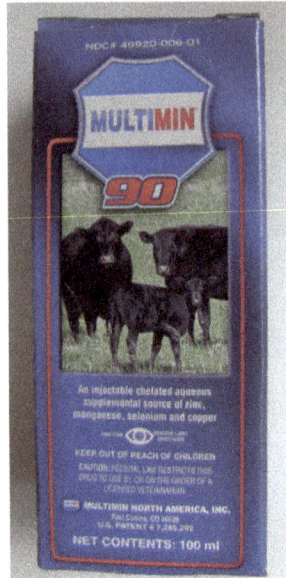

Image P19: *MultiMin, injectable mineral solution.*

For use in specific mineral deficiencies (Mn, Se, Cu, and Zn).

MultiMin USA
2809 East Harmony Road #190
Fort Collins, CO 80528
Phone: 970.372.2302
Fax: 970.631.8945

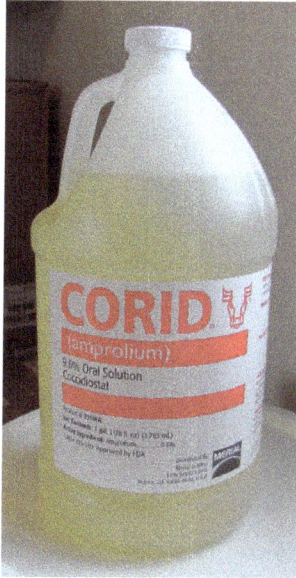

Image P20: *Corid liquid.*

Merck Animal Health U.S. Corporate Headquarters
2 Giralda Farms
Madison, NJ 07940
animal-health-communications@merck.com

Used for treatment against Coccidiosis spp. in calves. Corid can be purchased in powder form, which is more economical. Should be used within one week after mixing. Available in small packages for use in a few calves.

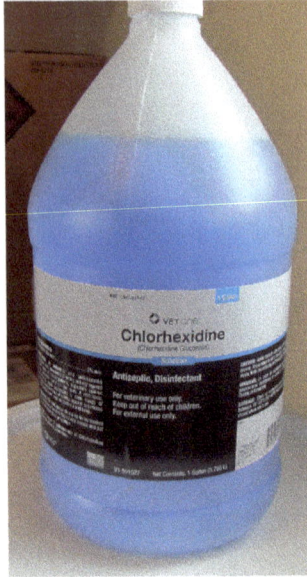

Image P21: *Chlorhexidine solution 2%. Chlorhexidine Gluconate is an antiseptic and antimicrobial disinfectant.*

Dilute 1 oz. of solution to 1 gal. clean water. Use as a cleaning solution for superficial cuts and abrasions.

Vedco Inc.
Saint Joseph Missouri
64507
(816)-238-8840

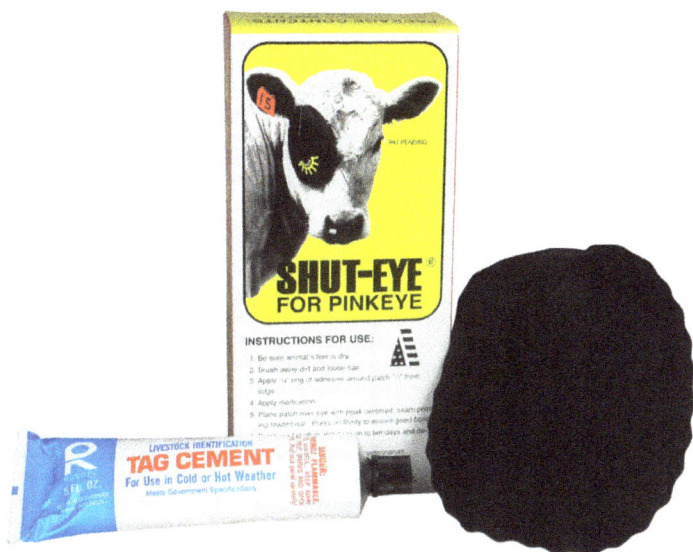

Image P22: *Shut-eye patches.*

American Animal Health, Inc.
P.O. Box 710 Wisner, Nebraska 68791
Phone: 402-529-3527
Fax: 402-529-3529
shuteye@pinkeye.com

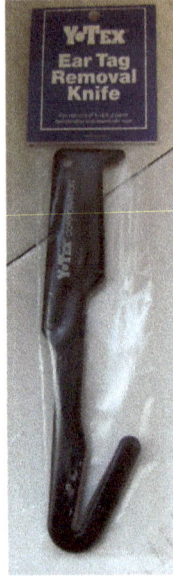

Image P23: *Y Tex Ear Tag Removal Knife.*

Y-Tex Corporation
1825 Big Horn Ave
Cody, WY 82414
(307) 587-1298

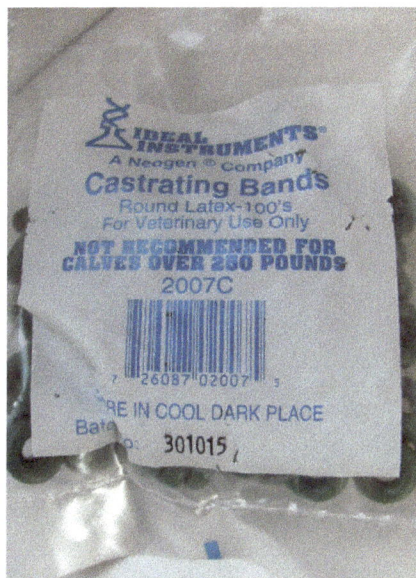

Image P24: *Elastrator castrating bands.*

Neogen Corporation
620 Lesher Place
Lansing, MI 48912 USA
Toll-free USA: 800-234-5333
Phone: 517-372-9200
Fax: 517-372-2006
www.neogen.com

Implants for calves

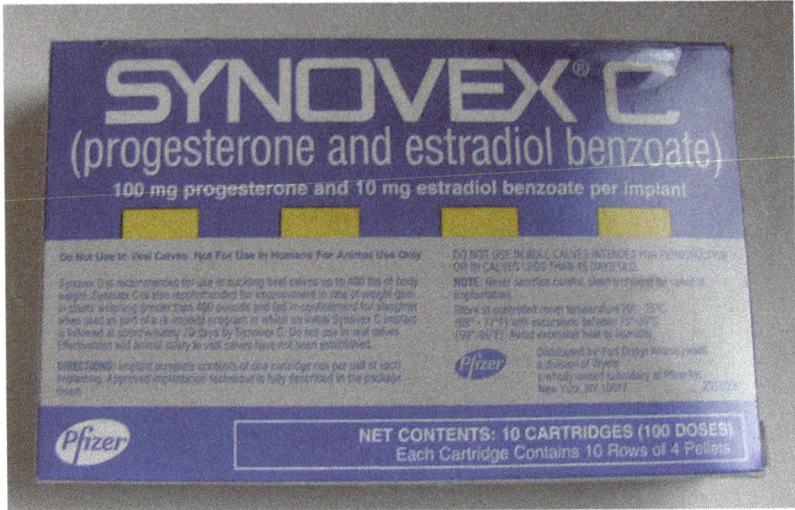

Image P25: *Synovex C calf implants.*

Zoetis Animal Health
1-888-ZOETIS-1 (or 1-888-963-8471)

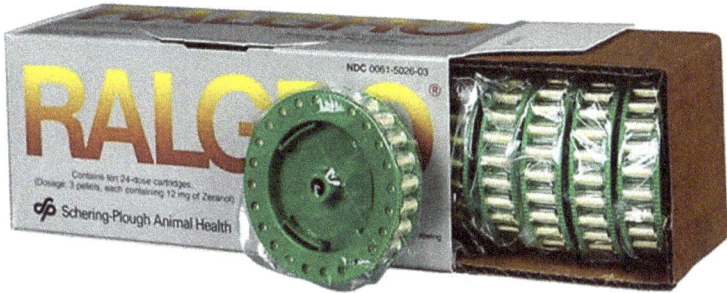

Image P26: *Ralgro calf implants.*

Ralgro is an anabolic agent which stimulates weight gain and feed efficiency in cattle. Each dose contains 36 mg (3 pellets) of Zeranol. Approved for suckling calves, growing beef cattle, feedlot steers and heifers, and replacement heifers between 1 month and weaning. Not cleared for use in heifers or bulls that will be used for breeding stock, lactating animals, or veal calves. No withdrawal period prior to slaughter.

Merck Animal Health U.S. Corporate Headquarters
2 Giralda Farms
Madison, NJ 07940
animal-health-communications@merck.com

Antibiotics compared

Trade name	Manufacturer	Generic name	Drug class
A 180®	Pfizer	danofloxacin	Fluoroquinolone
Baytril® 100	Bayer	enrofloxacin	Fluoroquinolone
Biomycin® 200	Boehringer-Ingleheim	oxytetracycline	Tetracycline
Draxxin®	Pfizer	tulathromycin	Macrolide
Excede®	Pfizer	ceftiofur	Cephalosporin
Excenel® RTU	Pfizer	ceftiofur	Cephalosporin
Liquimycin® LA200	Pfizer	oxytetracycline	Tetracycline
Micotil® 300	Elanco	tilmicosin	Macrolide
Naxcel®	Pfizer	ceftiofur	Cephalosporin
Nuflor®	Merck	florfenicol	Phenicol
Nuflor Gold®	Merck	florfenicol	Phenicol
Resflor Gold®	Merck	florfenicol & banamine	Phenicol & NSAID
Tetradure®	Merial	oxytetracycline	Tetracycline
Zactran®	Merial	gamithromycin	Macrolide

Table 16: *Antibiotics compared—name and drug class.*[91]

91. Data in all antibiotic comparison tables courtesy of Dr. John Maas, University of California, Davis, California, Veterinary Medicine Extension. Adapted for publication.

	M. hemolytica (BRD)	P. multocida (BRD)	H. somni (BRD)	Mycoplasma	Foot rot	Metritis	Pinkeye	E. coli scours	Woody tongue	Lepto pomona
A 180®	×	×								
Baytril® 100	×	×	×							
Biomycin® 200	×	×								
Draxxin®	×	×	×	×	×					
Excede®	×	×	×		×					
Excenel® RTU	×	×	×		×	×				
Liquimycin® LA200	×	×	×		×	×	×	×	×	×
Micotil® 300	×									
Naxcel®	×	×	×		×					
Nuflor®	×	×	×		×					
Nuflor Gold®	×	×	×	×						
Resflor Gold®	×	×	×	×						
Tetradure®	×	×	×		×	×	×	×	×	×
Zactran®	×	×	×							

Table 17: *Antibiotics compared—conditions treated.*

	Administration *	Duration of therapy	Withdrawal time
A 180®	SC	48 hrs.	4 days
Baytril® 100	SC **	3–5 days	28 days
Biomycin® 200	SC or IM	72 hrs.	28 days
Draxxin®	SC	7 days	18 days
Excede®	SC	6–7 days	none
Excenel® RTU	SC or IM	***	48 hrs.
Liquimycin® LA200	SC or IM	24–48 hrs.	28 days
Micotil® 300	SC	2 days	28 days
Naxcel®	SC or IM	24 hrs.	none
Nuflor®	SC or IM	24–48 hrs	IM 28 days; SC 38 days
Nuflor Gold®	SC	48 hrs.	44 days
Resflor Gold®	SC	48 hrs.	44 days
Tetradure®	SC or IM	7 days	28 days
Zactran®	SC	10 days	35 days

* *IM = intra-muscular, SC = subcutaneous*
** *Two dose rates for subcutaneous administration*
*** *3–5 days or 48 hours, depending on dosage and route of administration*

Table 18: *Antibiotics compared—administration, duration, and withdrawal.*

	Extra label use	Warnings and effects
A 180®	no	Not for use in dairy cattle
Baytril® 100	no	Not for use in dairy cattle
Biomycin® 200	yes	
Draxxin®	yes	Not for use in lactating dairy cows.
Excede®	not advised	Injection in the artery in the ear can kill cattle. Not for use in dairy cows.
Excenel® RTU	yes	
Liquimycin® LA200	yes	
Micotil® 300	not advised	Accidental injection in humans can be fatal.
Naxcel®	yes	
Nuflor®	yes	
Nuflor Gold®	yes	Not for use in lactating dairy cows.
Resflor Gold®	yes	
Tetradure®	yes	
Zactran®	yes	Not for use in lactating dairy cows.

Table 19: Antibiotics compared–extra label use and other notes.

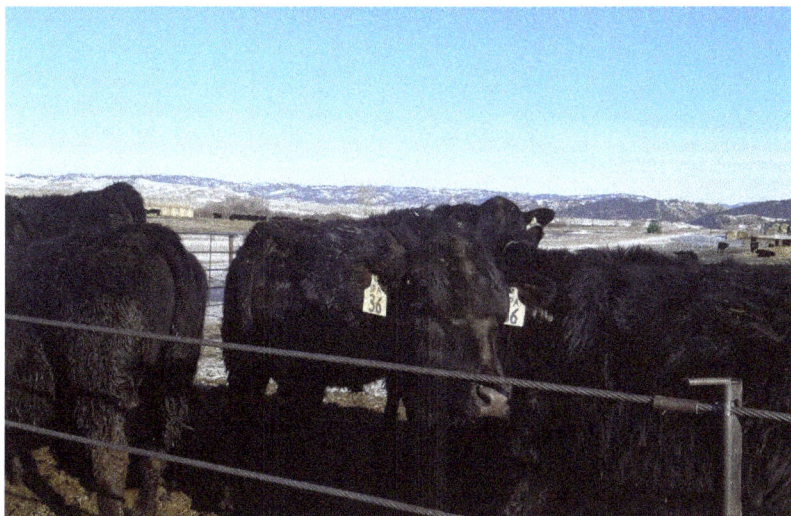

8

Supplemental

Future of Beef Production in the United States

There are many challenges in the future of the US beef cattle industry, but none greater than consumer demand, which will dictate profitability as in the past. As economic demands for production continue to increase, the recent expansion of the US cow inventory will result in lower prices in the future, resulting from a long-term supply outlook for more production.

An important key is US export demand world-wide, with increasing competition from countries like Russia and other countries where the costs of production are as low as one half of US production costs.

Global weather affecting forage and grain production pressures US beef production that was nearly immune decades before. Recent drought in the Southwest and the plains states in 2011 and 2012 forced the liquidation of entire cattle herds and produced 60-year lows in cow numbers. With the continued export demand, this created beef cattle prices only dreamed of by our parents, creating profits in 2014, especially in the cow-calf sector, never seen before in the history of US beef production. Prices were reported at $316 / cwt with 400–550 lb. steers, which resulted in greater than $1400 per head for weaned steer calves. This is double the number for 12 years before, and nearly 50% higher than two years before. This resulted in strong losses for feedlot operations, with losses of greater than $400 per head at harvest, as 80% of the total cost was in feeder calf prices rather than the usual 60–65%. This shows an excellent example of supply/demand and the volatility of the market. Future weaned calf prices will have to be lower for feedlots to offset losses from 2015–2016. Recommendations that reflect supply and demand are critical for future expectations and production goals that are much more important than ten years ago.

As of the writing of this book, prices for 2017–2018 have been more modest, with most steer prices in the $150–160/cwt price range. Economists predict this trend will continue for the next two to three years, as beef numbers continue to increase.

Even with lower prices, many experts predict good demand for future beef production world-wide, with the number one reason being simply that people like the taste of beef.

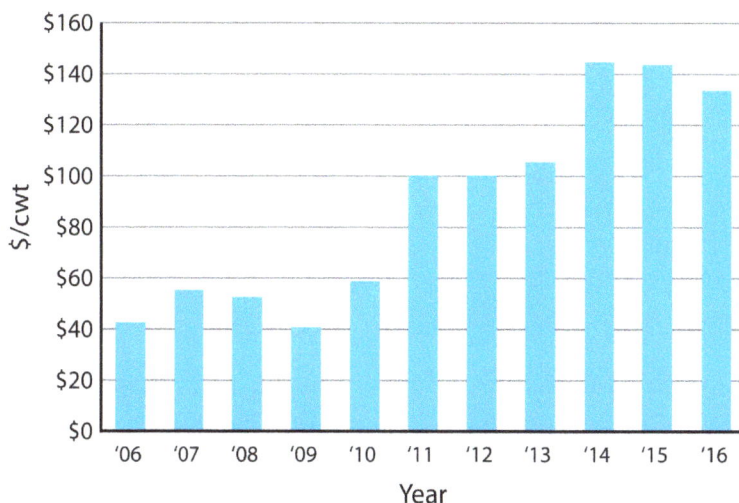

Figure 19: *Cattle futures, dollars per hundredweight, U.S. market.*

References and Citations

Berger, L. L., 1984. *Salt and Trace Minerals for Livestock, Poultry, and Other Animals*, Salt Institute, Alexandria, VA.

Cortese, V.S. 2009. Neonatal Immunology: Director Immunology Pfizer Animal Health, Simpsonville, Kentucky.

Cortese, V.S. 2009. Neonatal Immunology: Veterinary Clinics. *Food Animal Practice*, Volume 25. Number1. Pages 221–225, 2009.

Cortese, V.S., 2010. Annual Conference Proceedings, American Association of Bovine Practitioners, Albuquerque, NM, PG 82–84.

Engle T.E. 2001. *Effects of Mineral Nutrition of Immune Function and Factors that affect Trace Mineral Requirements of Beef Cattle*. Proceedings, The Range Beef Cow Symposium XVII, December 11–13, 2001, Casper, Wyoming.

Gropper, S.S., J.L. Smith, and J.L. Groff. 2007. *Advanced Nutrition and Human Metabolism*, Fifth Edition, Wadsworth, Belmont, CA.

Grotelueschen, D., et al., 2003. *Managing To Alleviate Calf Scours: The Sandhills Calving System*, Range Cow Symposium, Animal Science Department, University of Nebraska-Lincoln, Lincoln, NE.

Immunology and Infectious Diseases, P.O. Box 173610. Montana State University, Bozeman, MT.

Jutila, M., 2011, Meds 523. Immunology and Infectious Diseases, class notes.

Lane, M.V., M.S. Bulgin, and B.C. Anderson, 2000. *Treatment of sick Calves*, CL649, Cattle Producers Library, Cooperative Extension System Handbook.

Maas, J. 1968. *Cobalt Deficiency in Ruminants*. Large Animal Internal Medicine. 2nd ed. 908–911 National Research Council. 1984. Nutrient requirements of beef cattle, 6th ed., Washington D.C. National Academy of Sciences. 13–14.

National Research Council. 1985. *Nutrient requirements of sheep*, 5th ed. Washington D.C. National Academy of Sciences. 18–19.

National Research Council. 2005. *Mineral Tolerance of Animals*. Second Revised edition. 124–136.

Paterson, J. A., 2009. personal communication, ARNR 570, November 12, 2009.

Paterson, J. A., 2009. Beef/Cattle Extension Program, *What are the effects of calf health on feedlot performance?* www.animalrangeextension.montana.edu/articles/beef/Nutrition/calf/_health_profit.htm

Potter, T. *UK Vet*, Vol. 12, No 1, January 2007, The Royal Veterinary College, North Mymms, Hatfield, Herts. AL9 7TL.

Rodostits, O. M., C.C. Gay, K.W. Hinchcliff, and P.D. Constable. 2007, Veterinary Medicine, 10th ed. Saunders Elsevier, London UK.

Sager, R. B. 2000. Sage Trail Veterinary Calving Handout.

Sager, R. B. 2002. *Immune deficiency syndrome in nursing calves due to copper deficiency in the Williams herd*, Case report, 2002–143, Prepared for Pfizer Animal Health, Exton, PA.

Sager, R. B. 2007. *Immune System Function Deficiency in Nursing Beef*

Calves on Summer Pasture, Case report 2, Board Certification Paper, American Board of Veterinary Practitioners. Nashville, TN.

Smith, D.R., 2003. Proceedings, The Range Beef Cow Symposium XVIII, December 9–11, 2003, Mitchell, NE.

Smith, B.P., 2005. *Large Animal Internal Medicine*. 2nd ed. Mosby Publishing, USA. 541–547.

Smith, G.W. Editor, 2009. *Bovine Neonatology*. Veterinary Clinics Food Animal Practice, Volume 25, Number 1. March 2009.

Underwood, E.J. 1977. *Trace Elements in Human and Animal Nutrition*. 4th Ed. 132–139.

Underwood, E.J., and N. F. Suttle. 2004. *The Mineral Nutrition of Livestock*, 3rd ed. CABI Publishing, Wallingford Oxon OX10 8DE UK, 251–282.

White, B., Kansas State University, ABVP Symposium, St. Louis, MO, May 1, 2011. (2011; adapted from Smith, 2005).

Whittier, J.C., et al., 2000. *Preparing Calves for the Feedlot*, Cattle Producers Library, CL340, Cooperative Extension System Handbook.

Wildman, B. and D. Thomson, 2010. *Beef Production: Changes over the Years*, 43rd Annual Conference Proceedings, American Association of Bovine Practitioners, Albuquerque, NM, August 19–21, 2010, p 61–68.

List of Figures

List of Tables

List of Images

Product Images

Necropsy & Diagnostic Images

www.ingramcontent.com/pod-product-compliance
Lightning Source LLC
Chambersburg PA
CBHW042110220326
41598CB00071BA/7344